S0-BFC-732

Pharmacy
Practice Experiences
A Student's Handbook

Notices

The author and publisher have made every effort to ensure the accuracy and completeness of the information presented in this book. However, the author and publisher cannot be held responsible for the continued currency of the information, any inadvertent errors or omissions, or the application of this information. Therefore, the author and publisher shall have no liability to any person or entity with regard to claims, loss, or damage caused or alleged to be caused, directly or indirectly, by the use of information contained herein.

The inclusion in this book of any product in respect to which patent or trademark rights may exist shall not be deemed, and is not intended as, a grant of or authority to exercise any right or privilege protected by such patent or trademark. All such rights or trademarks are vested in the patent or trademark owner, and no other person may exercise the same without express permission, authority, or license secured from such patent or trademark owner.

The inclusion of a brand name does not mean the author or the publisher has any particular knowledge that the brand listed has properties different from other brands of the same product, nor should its inclusion be interpreted as an endorsement by the author or the publisher. Similarly, the fact that a particular brand has not been included does not indicate the product has been judged to be in any way unsatisfactory or unacceptable. Further, no official support or endorsement of this book by any federal or state agency or pharmaceutical company is intended or inferred.

Pharmacy Practice Experiences
A Student's Handbook

Paul J. Setlak, PharmD
Medical Services Coordinator
Abbott
Abbott Park, Illinois

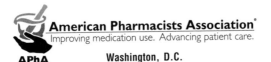

American Pharmacists Association®
Improving medication use. Advancing patient care.

APhA   Washington, D.C.

Acquiring Editor: Sandra J. Cannon
Editor: Paula Novash
Graphic Designer: Michele Danoff, Graphics By Design
Cover Design: Scott Neitzke, APhA Creative Services
Proofreader: Mary De Angelo
Indexer: Suzanne Peake
Editorial Assistance: Kellie Burton

© 2008 by the American Pharmacists Association
APhA was founded in 1852 as the American Pharmaceutical Association

Published by the American Pharmacists Association
1100 15th Street, NW, Suite 400, Washington, DC 20005-1707
www.pharmacist.com

All rights reserved

*No part of this book may be reproduced, stored in a retrieval system,
or transmitted in any form or by any means, electronic, mechanical,
photocopying, recording, or otherwise, without written permission from
the publisher.*

To comment on this book via e-mail, send your message to the publisher
at aphabooks@aphanet.org.

Library of Congress Cataloging-in-Publication Data

Setlak, Paul J.
    Pharmacy practice experiences : a student's handbook / by Paul J. Setlak.
        p. ; cm.
    Includes bibliographical references.
    ISBN 978-1-58212-114-7
  1. Pharmacy—Practice—Handbooks, manuals, etc. I. American
Pharmacists Association. II. Title.
    [DNLM: 1. Pharmaceutical Services—Handbooks. 2. Education,
Pharmacy—Handbooks. 3. Pharmacy—Handbooks. QV 735 S495p 2008]
    RS122.5.S48 2008
    362.17'82—dc22

                                2008003423

How to Order This Book
Online: www.pharmacist.com
By phone: 800-878-0729 (770-280-0085 outside the United States)
VISA®, MasterCard®, American Express® cards accepted

Dedication

This book, and my career, would not have been possible without the support of my parents and family who were all instrumental in providing me never-ending motivation during my years of education. To Kristy, my wife, for caring about us always.

To Dr. Mary Lee, my Dean while I was at Midwestern University – Chicago College of Pharmacy, who was always there to provide guidance and understanding.

Finally, to Dr. Michele Carbone, the most passionate, unwavering, and dedicated research physician I had the honor of working with for years.

Thank you all.

Medicine is the restoration of discordant elements; sickness is the discord of the elements infused into the living body.

—Leonardo Da Vinci
(Notes on Medicine Tr. 7; 853).

Table of Contents

Introduction

When we hear the word "pharmacist" we think of personal qualities such as thoroughness, compassion, and trust. From the moment that you put on your white lab coat, you will strive to uphold these high standards. In this way you help ensure that the profession of pharmacy, now your profession, will continue to be viewed as a steadfast source of health care provision, counseling, and empathy.

The role of the pharmacist is expanding rapidly as changing patient needs, federal oversight, and financial issues dominate the horizon. You have chosen a profession that is no longer viewed as simply "count, pour, lick and stick," but encompasses direct patient care and also the development of public policy and medical advances to improve and benefit patients' quality of life. Furthermore, as a pharmacist you are assured that your skills, knowledge, and analytical abilities will be valued by countless industries ranging from acute care hospitals to retail to investment banking and the legal sector.

If you are reading this book, you have probably already completed prerequisite courses and instruction and are well on your way towards obtaining your Doctorate in Pharmacy (PharmD). Many of you may have completed a Bachelor's degree prior to beginning your PharmD program. *Pharmacy Practice Experiences: A Student's Handbook* is designed to provide an easy, concise source for relevant information as it pertains to your education, your pharmacy practice experiences (PPEs), and your employment opportunities in various sectors.

In addition, the book covers material that is not often presented in depth at pharmacy schools. Many of these topics developed from situations I encountered during my own and my colleagues' training. For instance, as I worked with patients, I realized it would be helpful for pharmacy students to learn more about communication techniques and presentation skills. I also found myself using certain references over and over; some of them are included in the Appendix of this book.

You are likely looking forward to the vast array of PPEs available to PharmD candidates, as well as the large variety of employment opportunities. It is my hope that this Handbook will serve as a guide during your progression through these significant steps in your evolving career.

Paul J. Setlak, PharmD
Abbott Park, Illinois
January 2008

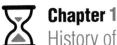

Chapter 1
History of the Pharmacy Profession

As you progress through your pharmacy practice experiences (PPEs) and embark upon your chosen career path, it is important to not only anticipate the exciting future of pharmacy but also to remember its fascinating history.

> φάρμακον
> Greek for "drug"

A Timeline of Pharmacy

From the beginning, humans have looked for substances and remedies to treat ailments. Early drawings portray how simple materials like mud and leaves were used for external medical problems such as cuts and irritations. How did ancient man determine which plants to apply topically as an early "bandage?" He employed the same analytical processes that you will use to decide whether a treatment is appropriate for a patient. The basic tenet by which you will select, adjust and determine appropriateness for a medication is simple—right disease, right drug, right dose.

> Right **DISEASE**,
> Right **DRUG**,
> Right **DOSE**

As man evolved, so did the profession of pharmacy. Writings and drawings from Babylonian civilizations dating back to 2600 B.C. demonstrated how specialized individuals were trained to recognize disease, suggest treatments, and spiritually nurture their patients. Across the world in the Far East, herbalists sought, tested, and recorded hundreds of natural remedies. Many of these are still well known today, including ginseng and ma huang (ephedra).

Around 2000 B.C., healers in the Egyptian empire compiled the "Papyrus Ebers." This collection of hundreds of prescriptions was a crucial resource for medical specialists and priests. North of Egypt, the Greek civilization was the birthplace to the world's first toxicologist—Mithridates. Not only was Mithridates an expert in identifying and making poisons, but he also successfully developed dozens of antidotes for commonly encountered overdoses and toxicities.

One individual truly stands out as the father of pharmaceutical compounding—the Roman Galen (130-200 A.D.). In addition to teaching and practicing medicine throughout the country, Galen was dedicated to combining various ingredients in order to individualize treatment for his patients. His recipes and methods were used throughout the Roman Empire and in a multitude of other civilizations around the world for almost 2000 years.

The complementary relationship between pharmacy and medicine was evident as far back as 300 A.D. when twin brothers Damian, a pharmacist, and Cosmas, a physician, worked together treating patients. So illustrious was their practice that the Christian church made them patron saints of medicine and pharmacy.

During the early Middle Ages, pharmacists shared their skills as they traveled to other parts of the world. The first pharmacies, or apothecaries, began to populate many busy cities in the European and Arabic regions. In addition, monasteries and other places of worship often maintained a supply of exotic medications, common remedies, and compounds for local inhabitants and patrons.

✕ A historical division between pharmacy and medicine occurred in the middle of the 13th century when Frederick II of Hohenstaufen issued an edict that separated and outlined responsibilities for each. Yet the commercial trading of medical products and philosophies between countries continued. The British were particularly large stakeholders in the trade of medical products and remedies. So large was Britain's medical industry that a company called "Master, Wardens and Society of the Art and Mystery of the Apothecaries of the City of London" was formed—the first organized society of pharmacists.

✕ The first organized hospital in Colonial America opened in Pennsylvania during the middle of the 18th century. The hospital was led by John Morgan, who was not only a pharmacist but also a physician. Morgan strongly supported each profession having specific roles and responsibilities.

✕ In 1821, the Philadelphia College of Pharmacy became the first pharmacy school on American soil, beginning the formal and consequently expanding profession of pharmacy. Three decades later, the American Pharmaceutical Association was formed to preserve the profession and its practices, provide guidance, and plan for the future.

✕ In the last century, both pharmacy and drug products grew at an astronomical rate. Multiple pharmacy schools opened, organizations specific to the needs of certain pharmacists were formed, and the discovery of novel treatments (such as antibiotics) came to fruition. The stage was set for the pharmacy profession to become an integral part of medicine.

Notes

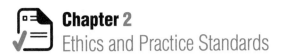

Chapter 2
Ethics and Practice Standards

Becoming a pharmacist means becoming a health care professional. By choosing pharmacy, you are accepting the great responsibility of taking part in the direct care and ongoing health of another person. From now on your first priority will be to act in the best interests of your patients.

The Code of Ethics for Pharmacists and the Oath of a Pharmacist (see Boxes 2-1 and 2-2) are key doctrines developed to address the ethical and fundamental issues of our profession. Although states may have individual pharmacy practice acts which discuss ethical expectations, these two documents provide all-inclusive guidelines that can be applied in any situation or location. As you pledge to uphold these tenets at your PharmD graduation, you may reflect upon the many ways pharmacy is intertwined in health care practices and the essential role you perform.

Box 2-1

Code of Ethics for Pharmacists
Preamble
Pharmacists are health professionals who assist individuals in making the best use of medications. This Code, prepared and supported by pharmacists, is intended to state publicly the principles that form the fundamental basis of the roles and responsibilities of pharmacists. These principles, based on moral obligations and virtues, are established to guide pharmacists in relationships with patients, health professionals, and society.

continued on page 6

Box 2-1 *continued from page 5*

I. A pharmacist respects the covenantal relationship between the patient and pharmacist.

Considering the patient-pharmacist relationship as a covenant means that a pharmacist has moral obligations in response to the gift of trust received from society. In return for this gift, a pharmacist promises to help individuals achieve optimum benefit from their medications, to be committed to their welfare, and to maintain their trust.

II. A pharmacist promotes the good of every patient in a caring, compassionate, and confidential manner.

A pharmacist places concern for the well being of the patient at the center of professional practice. In doing so, a pharmacist considers needs stated by the patient as well as those defined by health science. A pharmacist is dedicated to protecting the dignity of the patient. With a caring attitude and a compassionate spirit, a pharmacist focuses on serving the patient in a private and confidential manner.

III. A pharmacist respects the autonomy and dignity of each patient.

A pharmacist promotes the right of self-determination and recognizes individual self-worth by encouraging patients to participate in decisions about their health. A pharmacist communicates with patients in terms that are understandable. In all cases, a pharmacist respects personal and cultural differences among patients.

IV. A pharmacist acts with honesty and integrity in professional relationships.

A pharmacist has a duty to tell the truth and to act with

continued on page 7

Box 2-1   *continued from page 6*

conviction of conscience. A pharmacist avoids discrimi-
natory practices, behavior or work conditions that im-
pair professional judgment, and actions that compromise
dedication to the best interests of patients.

V. A pharmacist maintains professional competence.

A pharmacist has a duty to maintain knowledge and abilities as new medications, devices, and technologies become available and as health information advances.

VI. A pharmacist respects the values and abilities of colleagues and other health professionals.

When appropriate, a pharmacist asks for the consultation of colleagues or other health professionals or refers
the patient. A pharmacist acknowledges that colleagues
and other health professionals may differ in the beliefs
and values they apply to the care of the patient.

VII. A pharmacist serves individual, community, and societal needs.

The primary obligation of a pharmacist is to individual
patients. However, the obligations of a pharmacist may
at times extend beyond the individual to the community
and society. In these situations, the pharmacist recognizes the responsibilities that accompany these obligations and acts accordingly.

VIII. A pharmacist seeks justice in the distribution of health resources.

When health resources are allocated, a pharmacist is fair
and equitable, balancing the needs of patients and society.

American Pharmacists Association membership, October 27, 1994.

Box 2-2

Oath of a Pharmacist

- At this time, I vow to devote my professional life to the service of all humankind through the profession of pharmacy.

- I will consider the welfare of humanity and relief of human suffering my primary concerns.

- I will apply my knowledge, experience, and skills to the best of my ability to assure optimal drug therapy outcomes for the patients I serve.

- I will keep abreast of developments and maintain professional competency in my profession of pharmacy.

- I will maintain the highest principles of moral, ethical, and legal conduct.

- I will embrace and advocate change in the profession of pharmacy that improves patient care.

- I take these vows voluntarily with the full realization of the responsibility with which I am entrusted by the public.

American Pharmacists Association Academy of Students of Pharmacy/American Association of Colleges of Pharmacy Council of Deans (APhA-ASP/AACP-COD) Task Force on Professionalism, June 26, 1994.

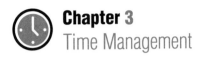

Chapter 3
Time Management

As pharmacists become more involved in multiple aspects of patient care, public policy, research, and consulting, managing time efficiently becomes a critical component of how effectively they are able to juggle their multiple responsibilities. Using your time well is especially important during PPEs where you will need to maintain a balance between patient care, disease state education, and individual research writing every day for more than a year. The ideas and strategies that follow will help you use your time productively.

In addition to managing your work time, you will find it helpful to schedule time for yourself to not only reflect on the week's activities, but also to "decompress." During this recharging time, you can pursue social activities with friends or family as well as pastimes you enjoy. If you push yourself to endure endless days without a break, you will suffer both mentally and physically—and so will your patients.

In addition, be sure to schedule some "flex" days or hours so if other issues come up (for example, an unexpected request from a physician requiring some research) you'll have ample time to work through those unexpected projects or tasks.

Tips for Structuring Your Day

Define Goals and Objectives with Your Preceptors.
Setting clear and defined goals and objectives for the entire course of your PPE is critical in helping you begin the process of time allocation. Once you have set your goals you

can better determine what proportion of your day you will spend on tasks such as disease state education, clinical skills, or presentations.

Develop a Daily Schedule.

For the most part, medical service teams follow a set schedule for patient rounding, educational series, in-services, and clinical presentations (see Box 3-1). Attempt to incorporate the projects that you and your preceptor agreed upon within this timeframe, because patient care should always come first.

Box 3-1

Sample Daily Schedule

6:30 am-9:00 am	Rounds
9:00 am-10:00 am	Patient case review
10:00 am-12:00 pm	Patient care
12:00 pm-1:00 pm	LUNCH
1:00 pm-3:00 pm	Patient care
3:00 pm-5:00 pm	Preceptor discussion

Develop a Methodology for Collecting Patient Information.

The saying "knowing is half the battle" is especially evident in very intensive PPEs, such as ICU or surgical. Construct a patient information sheet that you can carry around with you throughout the day, and update it as necessary. This care note should include some of the basic components you may need to refer to, including medications, laboratory values, recent procedures, allergies, etc.

Organize, Organize, Organize

Having excellent organizational skills is critical for successfully completing your PPEs, applying for jobs, and functioning effectively in the workplace. There are multiple organizational tools you can create to help you control information flow.

A simple example would be maintaining a file folder system for your PPEs (see Box 3-2). You can store the files in a cabinet or put them in a binder so that you can carry them with you to your various PPE sites. You might consider dedicating specific file folders to the following topics.

> Having excellent organizational skills is critical for successfully completing your PPEs, applying for jobs, and functioning effectively in the workplace.

Disease State Topics

Any disease state lectures and presentations that you discuss with your preceptor, fellow students, or any members of your medical team or staff should be placed into this file folder for future reference and updating.

Clinical Guidelines

Clinical guidelines are the basis of evidence-based medicine (EBM) and should always be referenced to determine the proper course of action in patient care. However, because medicine is an "individualized" practice, the guidelines may not always apply to your patient's specific situation. Not all patients present in the same way clinically, nor do they respond to therapy in an equal manner. Still, medical experts in their respective fields review guidelines rigorously and consistently. An excellent resource for finding clinical guidelines is the U.S. Government Guidelines Clearinghouse, which can be accessed at http://www.guidelines.gov.

This website is easily searchable and provides background on the guideline, information about its clinical applicability, individuals or society(ies) responsible for its publication, and a link to the full text itself.

Clinical Case Presentation(s)

Almost every PPE, whether it is retail, hospital, or managerial in nature, will require you to complete and present a case. Devoting a folder only to your cases will allow you to easily compile and retrieve information on your chosen topic. In addition, the contents of your case presentation folder can be copied and inserted in a "portfolio" that can be used to demonstrate your presentation skills at job interviews.

Patient Care Sheets

Patient-intensive PPEs, such as those based in an ICU or Emergency Department, usually have a high turnover of patients. Keep plenty of blank patient care sheets with you so you can easily find one when you need it.

Pharmacokinetics and Therapeutic Drug Monitoring

Always keep a copy of your institution-specific antibiogram.

Keeping lecture notes or sheets with a list of common pharmacokinetic principles and equations will make therapeutic drug monitoring (TDM) and assessment much easier. Compile a list of equations pertinent to the service that you are completing. For example, if you are on a pediatric ICU, you will need additional equations (i.e., clearance based on age) compared to the standard adult set.

And always keep a copy of your institution-specific antibiogram. Nothing can be more frustrating than trying to adjust antibiotic dosing and then realizing that it is useless because your specific hospital has a resistant bacterial strain.

Drug Information / Monograph

Your medical team, business colleagues, and patients will look to you for answers to drug information questions. In fact, many pharmacy programs require a PPE in drug information to enhance your knowledge and refine your research and analytical skills. Most will also require you to discuss a drug information question in writing and/or presentation format. Keep pertinent literature pertaining to your topic at hand along with a copy of the guidelines for proper reference citation and a lecture handout or guide on basic principles relating to biostatistics. You can use these for analyzing published literature and studies.

Administrative

Forms such as your schedule and contact information for your rotation site and pharmacy school's experiential office should be placed in this section. In addition, include copies of your pharmacy technician license, HIPAA statement, and a listing of your updated vaccination and immunization records. Also have records of any of your pertinent medical information, such as allergies, and contact information to use in the case of a medical emergency.

CV (Curriculum Vitae)

Update your CV regularly, including any clinical case presentations you completed, along with in-services, patient activities, publications, research, and pertinent projects. The CV is your "running tally" of what you have been able to accomplish during PPEs and helps employers review your training during the application process.

Box 3-2

In Your Folders....

Include these items relevant to your PPEs:

- Disease State Topics

- Clinical Guidelines

- Clinical Case Presentations

- Patient Care Sheets

- Pharmacokinetics and TDM

- Drug Information / Monograph

- Administrative

- CV

Notes

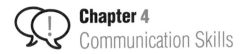

Chapter 4
Communication Skills

Communicating with patients and colleagues will be something you do regularly; it is an essential part of your pharmacy duties. By writing patient progress notes, chatting during patient rounds, or developing more formal presentations, you contribute to your health care team. And that contribution can be measured by how well you can impart your ideas and recommendations.

> Communicating with patients and colleagues is an essential part of your pharmacy duties.

Thinking about ways to become a better communicator and keeping tried-and-true ideas in mind will help you improve your skills.

Tips for Better Communication

Here are some techniques that you can incorporate into your practice.

Speak with Full Knowledge of the Topic and Expect the Unexpected.

Because it can be exciting to have medical team members depend on your advice, you may rush to answer their questions. But not fully researching an inquiry can be troublesome when individuals ask tangential questions.

Before you respond, thoroughly learn about your topic and also familiarize yourself with other subject matter that may relate to the inquiry. By being as well versed as possible you can anticipate some of the "odd" or rare questions that may arise. This will not only allow you to furnish a specific, accurate, and complete answer, but will showcase your analytical skills to the team and your preceptor.

Be Aware of the Characteristics of Your Audience.

When answering a question or providing an in-service to the nursing team or a medical unit, always be cognizant of your audience. The makeup of the group—examples include physicians, nurses, business leaders, or patients—will alter the way you deliver your message and/or recommendations. Whereas physicians and scientists may want to hear about a mechanistic approach to a problem or theories surrounding an issue, other professionals may simply want to know the clinical applicability of medical care.

Practice Makes a Difference.

Presenting a patient case to individuals who have more education and experience than you do may seem intimidating. By practicing beforehand, even if it is with family or friends, you can become comfortable with your subject matter and how you must adapt to audience interpretation and body language. For example, if you notice the majority seem uninterested during your disease state portion, consider incorporating more visuals to retain focus or eliminating some components since that segment could be too extensive.

In addition, practicing in advance will also show you how much time you are spending on specific sections and the overall presentation. Most communications with health care teams, businesses, and preceptors have a time restriction, ranging from a few brief moments to greater than 60 minutes. Knowing you are going to finish on time will help you feel at ease during your presentation. And staying within the time allotted also illustrates another key feature of your skill set: good organization.

Avoid Distracting Motions and Transition "Fillers."

Some individuals become "glued" to a podium or an object such as a pen and will unconsciously incorporate it into their body language. Fiddling with technical equipment, chewing on a pencil, or twisting a pointer constantly are some of the things you should avoid. Habits like these can easily distract the audience and make them lose track of your message, your knowledge, and ultimately, your presentation.

Although some individuals will stand in one place, others prefer moving around during their discussion. Whichever one you choose, make sure you are consistent and that it is appropriate. During rounds with your medical team you may want to stay in one place while speaking, whereas traversing the stage during a case presentation may allow the audience to focus directly on you and your message instead of just reading your PowerPoint slides.

If you take time to know, practice, and organize your information, the transitions between portions of your talk will sound very fluid. This should also help you avoid "fillers" such as "um," "and so," and "you know."

The Hierarchy System

All professions and industries employ some version of a hierarchy system in order to maintain a sequential method of reporting and delineating tasks. Pharmacy in various practice settings also has a hierarchical structure that should be recognized and adhered to.

Hierarchy in Hospitals

Pharmacy Director

Clinical and staff managers both report to the Pharmacy Director, who is responsible for overseeing the entire pharmacy department and its activities.

Centralized Staffing Managers

Centralized Staffing Managers supervise the centralized staffing pharmacists who primarily work within the pharmacy itself.

Clinical Manager

The Clinical Manager is usually the pharmacist who oversees the clinical programs of the pharmacy department and is in charge of the clinical staff.

Staff Pharmacists

Those pharmacists who do not directly provide clinical services, are not assigned to a specific medical service, or whose centralized duty is pharmacy dispensing services are referred to as staff pharmacists.

Clinical Pharmacists

Those pharmacists who directly provide clinical services, are assigned to a specific medical service for the majority of their time, or whose primary duty does not include pharmacy dispensing are referred to as Clinical Pharmacists.

Preceptor

The individual to whom you directly report and who is in charge of you as a PPE student is your Preceptor. The Preceptor might work in any of these pharmacy positions.

Pharmacy Technicians

Pharmacy Technicians are a crucial part of any hospital pharmacy and you should introduce yourself to them on the first day of your PPE. Technicians can be an excellent resource to show you the layout and intricacies of the pharmacy and how medications are stored, entered, prepared, dispensed, and accounted for.

In addition to the pharmacy department, there is also a typical hierarchy that should be adhered to when you are assigned to a medical team (see Figure 4-1).

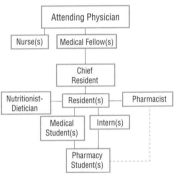

Figure 4-1.

Typical Hierarchy for a Medical Team in a Hospital Setting.

Hierarchy in Retail

Pharmacy Supervisors

Pharmacy Supervisors are in charge of a varying number of pharmacies contained within a predefined geographic region.

Pharmacy Manager

The Pharmacy Manager is in charge of the pharmacy operations at your specific retail PPE location; some of your days may be entirely spent with him or her.

Preceptor's Colleagues
Your preceptor's colleagues (fellow staff pharmacists) may also share responsibilities over your PPE.

Other Pharmacists
In addition to your preceptor and other staff pharmacists, you may also encounter part-time, floating, or "extra-board" pharmacists. These individuals are usually rotated through various stores depending on staffing needs and utilized to cover sick days and vacation time of the regular staff.

Preceptor
As in the hospital setting, the individual to whom you directly report and who is in charge of you as a PPE student is your Preceptor.

Pharmacy Technicians
Pharmacy Technicians are vitally important in the retail sector. Similar to their role in institutional settings, technicians can show you the layout and intricacies of the pharmacy and how medications are stored, entered, prepared, dispensed, and accounted for.

Resolving Communications Conflicts
Inevitably, you will encounter some conflicts that involve communication practices while on your PPEs. These situations may involve:

- The preceptor's or medical team's drug regimen choices.

- Timeframes set up for discussions and presentations.

- Company or institutional policies regarding a certain issue or practice.

- Personalities that differ on not only professional, but personal views.

- Professionalism, or lack thereof, in preceptors, medical staff, or co-workers.

- Favoritism, such as a preceptor listening to medical students or other team members instead of to you.

- Displays of disinterest or preconceived notions by preceptors.

- Inconsistencies or miscommunication on roles, responsibilities, and expectations.

It is very likely that you will experience one, if not more than one, of these situations during your PPEs and career. As you may recall from the Introduction, the number one rule for a practicing pharmacist is that the patient and his or her needs always come first. Therefore, it is imperative that any of these conflicts, usually involving communication, be identified and dealt with so as not to infringe on patient care. Although it may be intimidating to confront individuals such as your preceptor on these issues, not doing so will only complicate the situation(s) and make things worse as time progresses.

See Box 4-1 for some ideas and processes that will result in improved communications.

Box 4-1

Suggestions to Improve Communication

How should you deal with matters of conflict and mis-communications? Some ideas include:

- Identifying the situation as soon as it presents itself.

- Giving yourself time to decompress. Wait at least 24 hours to calm down and logically assess the problem(s).

- Documenting the circumstances surrounding the situation and any parties involved.

- Analyzing why this conflict may have occurred and what part you, your preceptor, and the work environment have contributed to it.

- Writing a summary of the event(s) and their progression.

- Requesting a sit-down discussion with your preceptor and possibly the other parties involved.

- Discussing with your preceptor, in an organized and coherent manner, the conflict, how you have been affected, and your suggested plan of action.

- Listening to your preceptor since he or she may have already dealt with a similar issue.

- Implementing an action plan and documenting it.

- Requesting a follow-up session with your preceptor to discuss the conflict's outcome.

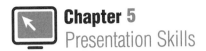

Chapter 5
Presentation Skills

Presentations are included in the majority of PPEs and often make up a good portion of your grade. Do not look at presentations as a way for preceptors and other supervisors to put you on the spot. Presentations provide a forum for you to showcase your pharmacy knowledge and skills.

> Presentations provide a forum for you to showcase your pharmacy knowledge and skills.

Types of Presentations

Journal Clubs

For a journal club presentation, you select an article or a topic that is relevant to your PPE and communicate it to your preceptor, colleagues, and fellow students. During hospital PPEs, many preceptors will give you freedom to select any peer-reviewed clinical article relevant to your medical service. In a retail or business setting, you may be asked to present an article or topic in line with the needs of the business or consumer (often on non-clinical subject matter). Nonetheless, there are some common attributes you should take into account when selecting and presenting a journal club, as shown in Box 5-1.

Box 5-1

Journal Club Presentation

When creating a journal club presentation, keep the following ideas in mind.

Clinical journal clubs should include a peer-reviewed, randomized, controlled, human clinical trial that is fairly recent (within 2 years of your presentation date) and published in a major reputable journal.

Avoid the following publications when selecting an article for your journal club:

- Case reports and series.

- Meta-analyses.

- Review articles.

- Editorials and commentaries.

- *In vitro* studies (unless your PPE requires it— i.e., drug company).

- Older studies (more than 2 years prior to your presentation date).

Be aware of how much time you are being given for your journal club (usually a range from 10 to 60 minutes).

Determine if your presentation will be informal (round-table discussion) or formal (PowerPoint required).

Always distribute a copy of the article and a summary of your analysis to the attendees.

Clinical Patient Case

Your clinical patient case presentation is the culmination of spending a tremendous amount of time caring for your patients on a medical service team. This formal discussion, oftentimes occurring during the last week of your PPE, should embody all the knowledge and expertise you have gained. As with journal clubs, there are some common attributes you should take into account when selecting and presenting a patient case, as shown in Box 5-2.

Box 5-2

Clinical Patient Case Presentation

Here are the steps involved in selecting and presenting a clinical patient case.

Select the patient whom you will model your presentation around as early as possible, which will give you ample time for preparation.

Be aware of how much time you are being given for your presentation (usually a range from 25 to 90 minutes).

Cover all pertinent areas of patient care during your case presentation, including:

- Disease state background.

- Patient history (medication history, prior admissions, allergies, etc.).

continued on page 26

Box 5-2

continued from page 25

- Drug information (mechanism of action, indications, dosing, monitoring, side effects).

- Patient progression from admission to discharge (or most current date).

- Your recommendation(s).

- Wider clinical applicability and how it relates to other possible cases in the future.

- Conclusion.

- References.

- Question and answer session.

PowerPoint Presentations

Microsoft PowerPoint is the standard format for students, professionals, and executives delivering formal presentations to an audience. The sooner you learn to use PowerPoint and become skilled in its capabilities, the easier it will be to develop, organize, and give strong presentations.

Here are some suggestions for incorporating PowerPoint presentations into your PPEs.

Use a Neutral Background with Minimal Distractions.

Studies have shown that the most effective color combination for PowerPoint presentations is the standard blue background with yellow text. Of course, it is important to make the presentation your own, but take into account fonts and colors that may prove to be too distracting or "fuzzy" for your audience. Finally, make sure that the font and type size you are using will be easily viewable by your audience.

Keep Number of Slides and Text to a Minimum.

Individuals have a tendency to put every single bit of information in their presentations. Be selective in what information you provide to your audience because you want them to be able to focus on you and what you are saying—not what is written. Furthermore, by limiting what is included on the slides, you will allow yourself to discuss tangential topics that add to the value of your topic or overall presentation. This also allows for leeway in terms of time constraints, giving you precious time to condense or expand on topics if you are running too slow or fast.

Choose your Slide Transitions and Animations Carefully.

Choose only a few slide transitions that are not distracting to the audience. Animations can be very useful when discussing mechanism of action or certain other aspects of a disease state. However, do not overuse them in slides where simple discussion or highlighting would suffice in making the same point.

Don't Forget Key Sections During the Presentation.

- **Objectives.** Allow the audience to immediately see what topics you will cover and how they relate to the patient that you will present.

- **Conclusion.** Presenting volumes of information is good, but being able to draw your own conclusions from the data, literature, and patient is superb.

- **References.** Your audience will appreciate you being able to properly cite and reference any and all literature that you used in preparation for your discussion.

Maintain Eye Contact.
The slides are a guide for you, but you need to impress the audience with your comprehensive knowledge and assessment of the patient and disease state management. If you just appear to be reading off your slides, the audience will become uninterested as they realize they could have read your presentation on their own.

Always Distribute Handouts.
Even though you are doing a formal verbal presentation, you should distribute a copy to the audience so that they can follow your talk, note comments on your slides, and discuss items for follow-up.

Notes

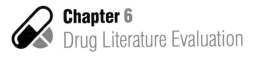

Chapter 6
Drug Literature Evaluation

Being able to evaluate and use drug literature effectively is an indispensable tool for a pharmacist. In order to properly assess the appropriateness of a medication regimen for a patient, analyze the post-marketing adverse events associated with a product, or find off-label indications for a particular drug, you must be able to read, analyze, critique, and reach conclusions based on published medical resources.

> You must be able to read, analyze, critique, and reach conclusions based on published medical resources.

Evaluating Drug Literature in Different Settings

You will need to evaluate drug literature in every PPE setting. Pharmacists in hospital pharmacies use drug literature evaluations for a multitude of activities, including P&T committees, patient care, research, protocol design, and medical safety. In retail pharmacies, corporate personnel, such as economic analysts who may also be pharmacists, constantly review for adverse event information and pharmacoeconomic data (sometimes this occurs in a department separate from the pharmacy) including cost comparisons between drug classes and generic versus brand formulations. Drug companies continually analyze newly published literature pertinent to their specific therapeutic areas and products in order to properly update their medical information for dissemination both externally (i.e., consumers and healthcare professionals) and internally (i.e., sales representatives and various divisions).

Sources for Review

Primary, secondary, and tertiary sources are used in drug literature review.

Primary Sources

Primary source literature forms the crux of drug information responses and therapeutic decisions. This type of literature consists of original research, usually published in peer-reviewed journals. One of the advantages of using primary sources is that they are published and updated frequently, often bi-weekly or monthly. Also, research manuscripts appear in print only after undergoing an intensive, in-depth review process. In order to gauge peer interest and gather commentary, many of these manuscripts are first presented as abstracts during conferences, symposiums, or seminars.

The most significant clinical studies tend to appear in the most prestigious and reputable journals. Journals which have a minimal "impact factor" (meaning the perceived importance of the journal to the medical community in a respective area of medicine) are likely to feature less significant information. For example, a major study that could have a wide effect on patient care would be unlikely to be found in a journal that has a high advertising-to-content ratio or is distributed without subscription fees.

It is important to note that review articles, even those from high-quality journals, are not considered primary literature because they are compilations of original research articles instead of results from new studies. Nevertheless, these articles can provide extensive background on disease states, practice guidelines, and clinical aspects of drug therapy.

Table 6-1 and Table 6-2 illustrate some of the types of literature and design variations you may encounter during your literature review.

TABLE 6-1. Examples of Primary Literature

Literature Type
▪ Original Experiments (*in vitro* and *in vivo*)
▪ Follow-Up Studies
▪ Case-Control Studies
▪ Cross-Sectional Studies
▪ Meta-Analyses
▪ Case Studies and Series
▪ Stability and Pharmacokinetic Studies
▪ Post-Marketing Surveillance Studies
▪ Economic Research

TABLE 6-2. Study Design Variations and Descriptions

Study Design	Description
Experimental	Investigate cause and effect relationships through interventions
Cohort (follow-up)	Observational experiments (no interventions)
Case-Control	Possible association between disease states and risk factor exposures
Meta-Analysis	Statistical analysis from compiled studies
Case Study and Series	Single or multiple patient observances (no interventions)
Post-Marketing	Adverse event manifestations after the release of a new medication or device
Economic	Evaluation of cost(s) associated with a therapy or device

Secondary Sources

Secondary sources generally consist of computerized databases that allow you to search for primary literature. One of the most commonly used is the NIH National Library of Medicine's PubMed at http://www.pubmed.gov. This searchable database is a regularly updated compilation of peer-reviewed articles that provide an abstract (if available), a link to the full text of the article, and also unique article identifiers and the complete citation in case the full-text link is not available. Users can search for published medical literature using keywords or MeSH terms that allow them to browse topics and subheadings for related articles.

Tertiary Sources

Tertiary sources include published materials such as textbooks. Although very comprehensive in nature, these sources may not be the most current; often they are updated too infrequently to keep up with the pace of advancing medical knowledge and pharmaceutical discovery. However, because these sources are usually incorporated in courses, lectures, and general reference, they can be excellent for background information, especially information related to disease states. Additionally, a majority of tertiary sources incorporate primary literature, providing you with a sampling of published studies that you can pursue in further detail.

Parts of a Research Study

Thousands of research study articles are published yearly in the biomedical sciences. You should assess every aspect of a study for appropriateness, quality, and conclusions using a step-by-step approach (see Figure 6-1).

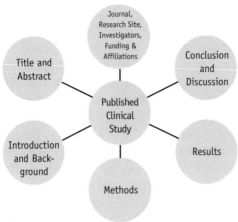

Figure 6-1.
Aspects of a Published Study that Must be Evaluated.

Journal

Knowing where the article was published will help you decide whether the information included is reputable and useful to you. Articles published in journals with a high advertisement-to-content ratio, no peer-review process, no subscription fees, and/or a low impact factor may not meet your requirements.

Research Site

A study conducted in a small community hospital with 50-100 beds may be less significant than an investigation done at a major academic institution with over 500 beds. Make sure you are aware of the type of facility where a particular study originated. In addition, many studies done outside of the U.S. should be examined to make sure different practice standards and varying drug formulations don't affect the results. And even if a drug used overseas is labeled "equivalent" to one in the U.S., you should investigate that claim by contacting the drug company.

Investigators

Check who conducted the study. If the researchers' credentials are in a specialty area markedly different from that covered in the article, you may want to investigate further. And when studies are largely funded by the pharmaceutical industry, you may consider possible bias or conflict of interest (although this is less true than in the past, due to greater federal and public scrutiny). Finally, having a biostatistician participating in the research study can be an indication that the results and conclusions are valid. (However, you may want to check whether the biostatistician is affiliated with the clinical researchers or another organization.)

Funding and Affiliation

Non-profit organizations such as the National Institutes of Health (NIH) or National Cancer Institute (NCI) are very reputable sources of research funds, as are colleges and universities. However, be aware that some funding organizations may support studies with outcomes favorable to their position(s).

Title and Abstract

It should be clear from the study's title and from the abstract what the investigation seeks to elucidate. In addition, these two components of a publication should not include any sort of bias favoring one outcome over another (an example would be a study titled "Drug X is superior to Drug Z").

Introduction and Background

The introduction and background should provide an adequate amount of information pertaining to the hypothesis being tested along with all pertinent disease state information. In addition, previous studies paralleling this investigation may be briefly discussed to inform the reader about what has already been done. Finally, and most importantly, the study objectives (possibly including primary and secondary outcomes) should be clearly and completely stated in these sections.

Methods

The methods portion of the study includes information on the design, patient population, protocol(s), and statistics employed. Even though a study may present pristine data and results, an unclear methods section may indicate that it is unreliable or compromised in some manner. Make sure that the methods section clearly discusses any ethical issues, along with the inclusion and exclusion criteria.

A study is only as good as the authors' definition of the patient population studied. Poor reporting of patient demographics, record-keeping, and/or inclusion and exclusion criteria may impede an article's quality. Whether or not there was a control, interventional variables, and randomization incorporation should also be clearly defined by the investigators. Finally, in addition to stating how data will be collected and analyzed, the authors should discuss what statistical methods will be employed to determine the significance of the data.

Results

First and foremost, the results section should define patient demographics and state how many patients from the original cohort were eliminated from the study, and for what reasons. (It sends a different message if patients are excluded for personal reasons versus due to adverse events associated with a new drug therapy.) Second, the results section has to answer every objective that was outlined in the beginning of the introduction and background. An objective left unanswered or skimmed through may be suspect. Results should be presented in a table or figure if possible, although some data may not work well in these formats. Finally, results should be defined as statistically significant or not, and if not, a possible explanation may be warranted.

Conclusion and Discussion

The final portion of the article should briefly recap the introduction and background of the study, and then summarize the methods and go into detail about the data and results. Any discrepancies in the patient population or results should be mentioned here by the authors. In addition, any study limitations that the authors have discovered during the course of the study should be mentioned. Finally, the investigators' conclusion(s) should be stated along with any future courses of action or studies to be considered on the topic.

Notes

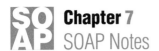

Chapter 7
SOAP Notes

You will become very familiar with SOAP notes during your PPEs. The SOAP format (the initials stand for Subjective, Objective, Assessment, and Plan) is the standard by which summative patient information is organized and presented to both pharmacy preceptors and other members of the health care team.

> The initials in **SOAP** stand for **S**ubjective, **O**bjective, **A**ssessment, and **P**lan.

Used by health care professionals ranging from physicians to nutritionists, the SOAP note is a concise and straightforward methodology of organizing relevant and important patient details into a succinct summary. This brief yet thorough synopsis should provide all pertinent information about a patient.

Importance of SOAP Notes

The type of information included in a SOAP note is listed in Box 7-1.

Box 7-1

What's in a SOAP Note?

Information covered in a SOAP note includes:

- Clinical presentation upon admission and progression pertaining to a patient's condition(s).

continued on page 38

Box 7-1

continued from page 37

- Significant medical events and drug-related problems.

- Pharmacotherapy, including patient's medications prior to admission.

- Proposed clinical course of action and any treatment modifications.

Patient charts can become very complex and contain volumes of information, so it is your responsibility to sort through the myriad of data and physician communications. Determining what is crucial from a pharmacotherapeutic and monitoring perspective will help foster a positive patient outcome.

Aside from reading patient charts, an ideal way for you to acquire critical information from your fellow health care professionals is by routinely attending patient rounds. Information that is presented by senior members of the medical team, such as the attending physicians and chief residents, may not be documented in the chart until later. Learning the most current patient information firsthand is invaluable in compiling your SOAP notes. And you can become a much more integral part of the medical team by rounding; it is an opportunity to incorporate many of your pharmacy-related suggestions into practice directly at the patient bedside.

> An ideal way for you to acquire critical information from your fellow health care professionals is by routinely attending patient rounds.

The SOAP Format

The typical SOAP note begins with a heading. This heading is very important to ensure consistent organization, especially when monitoring multiple patients who may have lengthy inpatient stays. Headers should include the date, time, medical service or unit name and patient room and/or initials, all formatted in accordance with federal and institutional HIPAA regulations.

Before developing and presenting a patient SOAP note, you must be able to differentiate between the individual components of it to determine exactly what patient information belongs in which section. The four detailed parts of a SOAP note follow.

Subjective

The Subjective section includes information about the present illness that is presented to health care professionals by the patient. This part of the note should clearly state the patient's age, sex, race (if pertinent; some medications have shown better efficacy in specific ethnic groups), chief complaint (CC) and any relevant review of systems (ROS) findings. The CC states exactly why the patient has sought medical help or the reason for being admitted to the hospital. A question to consider is, What are the patient's complaints?

The ROS component should list any pertinent signs or symptoms the patient has experienced directly related to the CC. A question to ask might be, What are the signs or symptoms of the patient's condition?

The Subjective portion also contains patient information that is considered non-reproducible or difficult to quantify, unlike laboratory values which are reported in the Objective section. It should also include the patient's social history (amount and frequency of alcohol, tobacco, and illicit drug use) and family history (parents, children and siblings), which can directly affect patient care and treatment approaches.

Additionally, you should also mention medications the patient was on prior to admission and any related past medical history (PMH). Although the drug history and PMH will be abbreviated in your SOAP note, it is essential to obtain an extremely thorough drug history for each patient in order to associate each prescribed medication with a concurrent true indication. With the increasing costs of health care and third party stringency, it may also be beneficial for you to gather information about the patient's current employment, insurance, and financial status and include it. Oftentimes, a similar medication that costs significantly less can be as efficacious as newer and more expensive therapies.

An example of the Subjective portion of the SOAP Note can be found in Box 7-2.

Objective

The objective portion of your SOAP note, generally the longest, states results and information gathered from the physical exam, laboratory tests, imaging, and any other exploratory procedures. This section always begins with the patient's vital signs (VS), which consist of five components:

- Temperature (°C)
- Heart Rate (HR)
- Respiratory Rate (RR)
- Blood Pressure (BP)
- Pain (rated on a scale of 0-10)

After listing the VS, it is necessary to record the patient's height (in inches) and actual body weight (in kg), especially

Box 7-2

Sample Subjective Section of a SOAP Note

TW is a 23-year-old male transferred to the burn service from Shreveport Medical Center after complaining of intensifying pain (7-9/10) from sustained scald burns to his right lower extremity. Patient also complains of difficulty moving his right lower extremity.

Patient denies alcohol or illicit drug use and states that he has smoked ½ pack per day of cigarettes for a little over 4 years now. TW is a single male living in suburban Illinois with his two parents. Currently, the patient is unemployed due to his diagnosed neurological degenerative disorder, leukodystrophy.

Current medications	Indication
1. Citalopram (Celexa®) 20 mg QDay (x6 years)	Major depressive disorder
2. Baclofen (Kemstro) 20 mg QDay (x3 years)	Spasticity – Leukodsytrophy

Allergies: Penicillin, Iodines

noting any significant changes in body weight. These two measurements are of paramount importance to the pharmacy staff when calculating doses for many medications and renal function. Secondly, when writing details about the patient's physical exam (PE), only include pertinent positive and negative aspects of the examination, not every single physical assessment. Keep in mind that what is considered to be pertinent in the patient's physical exam depends on which PPE you may be completing. For example, a PPE in a neurological ICU will focus on different aspects of the physical exam than would a PPE conducted in an anticoagulation clinic.

Following the physical exam details in your SOAP note are both the completed and pending laboratory results for the patient. Those laboratory values which are time-specific (such as drug level monitoring) require you to note when the specimen (usually blood) was drawn from the patient. In addition, it is imperative that you remember to specify exactly if and when the test result was labeled "final," since many "preliminary" results can present erroneous findings. The chem-7 and CBC panels are the most commonly ordered tests on patients because they can provide a vast amount of information on the patient's status and differential diagnosis (see Chapter 9 for more information). Results can be easily reported in the SOAP note by the commonly used "Fence and Fork" and "X" figures (see Figures 7-1 and 7-2) for the Chem-7 and CBC panels, respectively.

Na (Sodium)	Cl (Chloride)	BUN (Blood Urea Nitrogen)	Glu (Glucose)
K (Potassium)	HCO_3 (Bicarbonate)	SCr (Creatinine)	

Figure 7-1. Chem-7 Fence and Fork.

Finally, any other laboratory (i.e., cultures, ABG), imaging (i.e., X-rays, CT scans), or procedural results (i.e., EKG, endoscopy) that are also deemed relevant should be included in a logical and orderly manner after these two important panels.

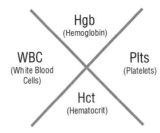

Figure 7-2. CBC X.

Although the Objective section of the SOAP note (see Box 7-3) is generally the lengthiest, it is important to reemphasize that your note has to be a succinct summary, especially focusing on information and results that primarily relate to the patient's pharmacotherapy.

Assessment

The Assessment portion of your SOAP note should sequentially address all the major problems with the patient that are supported by the Subjective and Objective sections, beginning with the most urgent issue. You might ask yourself, What are the medical and drug-related issues with this patient?

This section should also briefly discuss how the patient is doing and what has changed from the previous day, which can be deduced from the physician progress notes in the patient chart or during patient rounds. Be aware that it is not within your scope of practice to make a patient diagnosis, but you are well within your capacity to directly identify any pharmacotherapeutic issues.

The Assessment can be one of the most difficult components of the SOAP note to prepare (especially from a pharmacy perspective) since it requires you to analyze all of the Subjective and Objective data to formulate a ranked problem list.

Box 7-3

Sample Objective Section of a SOAP Note

PE:
VS $\underline{T}$ 37.2   **HR** 84   **RR** 18   **BP** 132/76 **PAIN** 7-9/10
       HT 66 in **ABW** 58 kg **IBW** 63.8 kg **BSA** 1.64 m² **CrCl** 105 mL/min

GEN slow dysarthric and spastic speech   **MUSC** weak ROM (extremities)
HEENT PERRLA, MMM   **SKIN** pink, warm and dry
RESP normal air entry, (-) distress, cough **NEURO** AOx3, CN 2-12 GI,
CARD RRR, no murmur   decreased tongue ROM, mild
GI (+) BS, NTND   right facial droop, lateral gaze
GU Not applicable   **PSYCH** kempt appearance,
                                                at times antisocial

LABS:
9/7/07 (Urine)

Color Yellow	**Clarity** Clear	**pH** 6.5	**Protein** (-)
Blood (-)	**Glucose** (-)	**Ketones** (-)	**Bilirubin** (-)
Urobilinogen <2.0	**Nitrites** (-)		**Leukocytes** (-)

9/9/07

Na 138	**Cl** 106	**BUN** 7	**Glu** 120
K 3.6	**CO$_2$** 24	**SCr** 0.9	
Ca 8.2 (1.12)	**Phos** 3.3	**Mag** 1.9	**pH** 7.39
PLT N/A	**WBC** N/A	**RBC** 4.26	
Hgb 12.7	**Hct** 38.1	**MCV** 89.4	

9/10/07

Na 142	**Cl** 104	**BUN** 5	**Glu** 91
K 4.4	**CO$_2$** 29	**SCr** 0.9	**CrCl** 105 mL/min
Ca 9.0 (1.23)	**Phos** 4.3	**Mag** 2.3	**pH** 7.32
PLT N/A	**WBC** N/A	**RBC** 4.64	
Hgb 13.9	**Hct** 40.6	**MCV** 87.5	

Daily Recorded I/O			
Date	**I/O (mL)**	**Date**	**I/O (mL)**
9/4/07	1380/230	9/8/07	1200/1400
9/5/07	3000/3300	9/10/07	2900/1200
9/6/07	2500/1800	9/11/07	1000/2300
9/7/07	1900/2000	9/13/07	1200/600

Plan

The last part of your SOAP note, oftentimes grouped together with the Assessment, is the Plan. The Plan is your opportunity to discuss what you would recommend be done, from a pharmacotherapeutic standpoint, to remedy each medical problem you formulated in the Assessment. This section should include any medication additions, changes, or discontinuations, as well as therapeutic alternatives deemed to be more appropriate. The Plan portion also covers necessary monitoring parameters, patient education, and follow-up instructions.

Examples of the Assessment and Plan sections of a SOAP Note can be found in Box 7-4.

Box 7-4

Sample Assessment and Plan Sections of a SOAP Note

PROBLEM LIST:
1. Lower right extremity burn wound (4.5% TBSA 2nd/3rd degree)
2. Drug (anesthetic) sensitivity
3. Idiopathic leukodystrophy (spasticity)
4. Major depressive disorder

PATIENT PROGRESSION:
9/3   Patient admitted to the LUMC burn service from Rush-Copley Medical Center. Standard labs are ordered (CMP, CBC) and are WNL. Patient appears tired, but rates pain as 7-9/10. Burn assessment is described as being a 5% TBSA (second/third degree) scald burn to the right anterior lateral lower leg, foot and circumferentially on toes.

continued on page 46

Box 7-4

continued from page 45

Patient is also agitated and disinterested when talked to numerous times.

R_x: Bisacodyl 5 mg tablet PO QHS (given x1)
Docusate sodium 100 mg capsule PO BID (given x1)
Nicotine 21 mg patch QDaily (given x1)
Zinc sulfate 1 mg tablet PO BID (given x1)
Baclofen 20 mg tablet PO QHS (given x1)
Hydrocodone/APAP 7.5-500 mg 2 tablets
    PO Q4H PRN (given x1)
SSD 1 container apply to wounds BID (given x1)

9/4 Patient VS are stable. No acute events overnight. Pain is still within the 7-9 range, per patient and family members, during wound care. Difficult to understand patient due to speech impairments.

R_x: Bisacodyl 5 mg tablet PO QHS (given x1)
Docusate sodium 100 mg capsule PO BID (given x2)
Glutamine 20 g packet PO BID (given x1)
Morphine 4 mg injection BID (given x3)
MV 5 mL oral solution PO QDaily (given x1)
Nicotine 21 mg patch QDaily (given x1)
Vitamin C 10 mL liquid PO QDaily (given x1)
Zinc sulfate 1 mg tablet PO BID (given x2)
Baclofen 20 mg tablet PO QHS (given x1)
Hydrocodone/APAP 7.5-500 mg 2 tablets
    PO Q4H PRN (given x4)
SSD 1 container apply to wounds BID (given x3)
Morphine 30 mg IR tablet PO BID PRN (given x2)

continued on page 47

Box 7-4

continued from page 46

9/5 Patient VS are stable. No acute events overnight. Pain is being controlled much better, per patient's family members. Surgical assessment determines that appropriate course of action includes split-thickness skin grafts from left leg. Surgical date set to be 9/8. Psych consult recommends continuing with previous anti-depressant therapy, citalopram 20 mg PO QHS.

   R_x: Bisacodyl 5 mg tablet PO QHS (given x1)
      Citalopram 20 mg tablet PO QHS (given x1)
      Docusate sodium 100 mg capsule PO BID (given x2)
      Glutamine 20 g packet PO BID (given x1)
      Morphine 4 mg injection BID (given x3)
      MV 5 mL oral solution PO QDaily (given x1)
      Nicotine 21 mg patch QDaily (given x1)
      Vitamin C 10 mL liquid PO QDaily (given x1)
      Zinc sulfate 1 mg tablet PO BID (given x2)
      Hydrocodone/APAP 7.5-500 mg 2 tablets
        PO Q4H PRN (given x3)
      SSD 1 container apply to wounds BID (given x3)
      Morphine 30 mg IR tablet PO BID PRN (given x2)

9/8 Patient VS are stable. No acute events overnight. Surgical grafting occurs without complications. No allergic reactions were noted during procedure. Total grafting consisted of 700 cm^2.

   R_x: Bisacodyl 5 mg tablet PO QHS (given x1)
      Citalopram 20 mg tablet PO QHS (given x1)
      Docusate sodium 100 mg capsule PO BID (given x2)

continued on page 48

Box 7-4

continued from page 47

> Glutamine 20 g packet PO BID (given x1)
> Morphine 4 mg injection BID (given x3)
> Morphine 30 mg CR tablet PO Q12H (given x1)
> MV 5 mL oral solution PO QDaily (given x1)
> Nicotine 21 mg patch QDaily (given x2)
> Ondansetron 4 mg PO Q8H PRN (given x1)
> Vitamin C 10 mL liquid PO QDaily (given x1)
> Zinc sulfate 1 mg tablet PO BID (given x2)
> Hydrocodone/APAP 7.5-500 mg 2 tablets
>   PO Q4H PRN (given x2)
> SSD 1 container apply to wounds BID (given x2)
> Cefazolin 1g IVPB (given x1)
> $D_5W_{1/2}NS$ with 20 mEq K (83mL/h) (given x1)

9/9-13   Patient VS are stable. No acute events. Skin grafts are taking very well with pigmentation emerging. No signs of rejection or infection are present. Plan is to transfer patient down to 5th floor rehabilitation unit for PT/OT. SSD dressings are to be continued on the toes and foot, while bacitracin dressings are to be applied to the anterior lateral lower portions of the legs.

   R_x: Bisacodyl 5 mg tablet PO QHS (given x1)
> Citalopram 20 mg tablet PO QHS (given x1)
> Docusate sodium 100 mg capsule PO BID (given x2)
> Glutamine 20 g packet PO BID (given x1)
> Morphine 4 mg injection BID (given x3)
> Morphine 30 mg CR tablet PO Q12H (given x1)
> MV 5 mL oral solution PO QDaily (given x1)

continued on page 49

Box 7-4

continued from page 48

> Nicotine 21 mg patch QDaily (given x2)
> Ondansetron 4 mg PO Q8H PRN (given x1)
> Vitamin C 10 mL liquid PO QDaily (given x1)
> Zinc sulfate 1 mg tablet PO BID (given x2)
> Hydrocodone/APAP 7.5-500 mg 2 tablets
>   PO Q4H PRN (given x2)
> SSD 1 container apply to wounds BID (given x2)

REHABILITATION ORDERS:
9/14 Patient was discharged at 1430 from the burn service to the rehabilitation floor to commence OT/PT. Goals include improving range of motion in extremities, with a focus on the right leg, foot and toes involved in the thermal injury. Additionally, speech and oral training will be instituted to improve communication and eating skills. Psychology and social work will continue with both patient and family on known issues. Continuation of all prior inpatient medications is warranted, along with oral baclofen for spasticity. Pain medication will be continued as oral morphine or hydrocodone/APAP, with the possibility of switching to oxycodone if pain becomes significantly worse.

DRUG THERAPY RECOMMENDATIONS:
1. According to the standard burn service protocol, all fluids and supportive treatments were appropriate for this patient's thermal injuries. Additionally, twice daily dressing changes were appropriate due to the severity of his TBSA. Pain was controlled as best as possible

continued on page 50

Box 7-4

continued from page 49

during the patient's hospitalization, although it was difficult to communicate sometimes with the patient due to his speech impairments.

2. Surgical intervention proceeded without complications. Anesthetic sensitivity as described by patient's family was not encountered. Skin grafts took very well to the areas on his lower extremities and there were no apparent signs of infection or rejection.

3. Leukodystrophy-related spasticity was controlled with baclofen as ordered by overseeing neurologist, although the condition has been termed as being "in remission" by both physician and family.

4. Anti-depressant medication, citalopram, was appropriate and continued throughout burn service stay and subsequent rehabilitation.

5. Rehabilitation consisting of PT/OT and speech training is appropriate for this patient considering his neurological condition and long-term need for improvement.

6. Pharmacist recommends continuing pain medication as needed on an outpatient basis, preferably an immediate release formulation for any breakthrough pain. Furthermore, suggest follow-up with primary care physician to assess healing of burn wounds and continuation of both baclofen and citalopram based on response and presentation of adverse events.

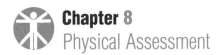

Chapter 8
Physical Assessment

In addition to taking part in the management of medication regimens, many pharmacists are assisting in the general clinical assessment of patients. A growing number of ambulatory and retail clinics and collaborative practices are among the settings for PPEs involving physical assessment.

> Many pharmacists are assisting in the general clinical assessment of patients.

Patient Evaluation

When assessing a patient's condition, you will consider a number of factors. Here are some key aspects of patient appearance and vital signs to evaluate.

Age
The patient should resemble a typical person of his or her years.

Skin
The color of an individual's skin and blemishes and/or lesions may suggest some sort of pathology. For instance, pallor might indicate infection. Jaundice, which is a yellowing of the skin, suggests a liver or gallstone pathology. Skin lesions that are peculiar in shape, size, or color should also be noted.

Facial Features
Individuals' faces should have a symmetrical appearance, without any visible or obvious drooping or abnormal shapes. Additionally, an individual whose face presents a "flat effect" (characterized by lack of expression, staring into space, not

responding to questioners) may be suggestive of depression or a neurological deficit.

Consciousness
The person you are assessing should be alert, awake, and oriented to time and place. Asking a patient simple questions such as his or her name, location, and the current date can immediately clue you into any possible mental status changes or neurological pathologies.

Acute States
Looking at the individual should help you identify any signs or symptoms of acute stresses. Some events you should pay close attention to include shortness of breath (SOB), wheezing, and holding or covering certain body areas.

Nutrition and Weight
Healthy individuals should be within the suggested height and weight ranges for their ages and genders. Any significant deviations should be noted and conveyed to the physician or nurse practitioner for follow-up. Of special concern are those individuals who appear cachectic (very thin or emaciated; this can be a characteristic of chronically wasting diseases).

Calculating the patient's body mass index (BMI) may also be beneficial. However, you must take into account the person's muscle mass—healthy individuals with a high amount of muscle and low body fat have sometimes been characterized as having a dangerously high BMI (see Table 8-1). Finally, ask the patient about any significant changes in weight or eating habits, both of which may suggest a concurrent disease process.

TABLE 8-1. BMI Classification

BMI	Classification
<18.5	Underweight
18.5 – 24.9	Healthy Weight
25 – 29.9	Overweight
30 – 34.9	Obese (mild)
35 – 39.9	Obese (moderate)
≥40	Obese (severe)

Behavior

The patient should be responsive to your questions and physical assessment. Any odd behavior, such as losing attention quickly or being combative, should be documented.

Mobility

Allow the individual to stand up and move around both in a straight line and in a circle in order to gauge ambulatory status and any obvious gait or balance issues. Be very careful if the patient seems off balance and remain with him or her at all times.

Vital Signs

Historically, a patient's vital signs have consisted of temperature, heart rate, blood pressure, and respiratory rate. Because of the health care system's push to make sure that individuals are being treated appropriately for pain, the fifth vital sign now commonly included is an evaluation of the intensity of pain that a patient is experiencing.

Temperature (T)

The normal range for adults is 36.4-37.2°C. Due to diurnal variances, exercise, age, and hormones, a person's body temperature can deviate safely within 1°C. This measurement is especially useful in helping determine an ongoing infectious process, although elevated temperature may not be present in elderly patients. Temperature can be measured by employing one of the following methods, using a digital thermometer.

Oral
The most commonly used technique; it is both convenient and accurate. Normal oral temperature is 37°C.

Rectal
This method is especially useful for infants, children, and patients who have difficulty with an oral access route or are intubated. Furthermore, rectal measurement is the most accurate in obtaining a person's core body temperature. Normal reading in adults is 37.5°C.

Axillary (armpit)
This route can be used in both adult and pediatric patients. The normal reading for an axillary temperature is 37.7°C.

Tympanic (ear)
Reading a patient's temperature via the ear canal requires a digital thermometer with a probe. The advantages of this method include ease of use and obtaining a reading in as little as 2 seconds.

Pulse (HR)
The normal range is 60-100 beats per minute (bpm) in healthy individuals (see Table 8-2). A person's heart rate can vary due to diurnal variances, exercise, age, and hormones, resulting in a wide range within normal limits. Measurement of heart rate is especially useful in helping determine cardiovascular events (as well as numerous other pathologies). In

addition to the number of beats, you should assess the strength of each beat and any abnormal rhythms that may suggest an arrhythmia.

If the patient is not on a heart rate monitor, you can check his or her heart rate by placing the pads of your first and second fingers on the surface of the wrist, medially to the radius. Press down (not so firmly as to cause occlusion) and you will begin to feel a pulse. Count the number of beats over 15 seconds and multiply that number by four to determine the beats per minute. If the pulse is very rapid, slow, or irregular, you will obtain a more accurate reading by counting the number of beats over 30 seconds and multiplying by two.

> The term for a heart rate over 100 bpm is tachycardia.
> The term for a heart rate under 60 bpm is bradycardia.

The term for a heart rate over 100 bpm is tachycardia. The term for a heart rate under 60 bpm is bradycardia.

TABLE 8-2. Normal Heart Rate (HR) for Various Age Groups

Age (y)	HR (bpm)
Newborn and up to 1 year	70-170
1-6	75-160
6-12	80-120
Adult and >65	60-100

Respiratory Rate (RR)

Normal range is 12-20 breaths per minute in healthy individuals (see Table 8-3). Due to diurnal variances, exercise, age, and hormones, a person's respiratory rate can vary, so the range of normal limits is wide. Measurement of respiratory rate is especially useful in helping determine a respiratory event or infectious process, in addition to other pathologies. The strength or weakness of an individual's breaths can also be significant for further investigation.

If the patient is not on a ventilator or monitor, his or her respiratory rate is normally assessed by observing the chest moving up and down, with one complete movement in both directions comprising one respiratory rate. Since respirations usually occur much less frequently than pulse over the course of a minute, respiratory rate should be assessed for a minimum of 30 seconds and multiplied by two, or evaluated for a full minute.

> The term for a respiratory rate greater than 20 breaths per minute is tachypnea. The term for a respiratory rate of less than 12 breaths per minute is bradypnea.

The term for a respiratory rate greater than 20 breaths per minute is tachypnea. The term for a respiratory rate of less than 12 breaths per minute is bradypnea.

TABLE 8-3. Normal Respiratory Rate (RR) for Various Age Groups

Age (y)	RR
2-6	21-30
6-10	20-26
12-14	18-22
Adult and >65	12-20

Blood Pressure (BP)

BP is considered to be normal if it is less than or equal to 120/80 in healthy individuals (see Table 8-4). Due to diurnal variances, exercise, age, diseases, and hormones, a person's blood pressure can vary. The "gold standard" for measuring blood pressure is through a catheter, but the sphygmomanometer is the most commonly employed device that is used in an outpatient setting. Measurement of blood pressure is especially useful in helping determine a cardiovascular issue in patients, in addition to other pathologies.

In order to manually take an individual's blood pressure, you must practice multiple times to gain confidence and master the technique. This process is outlined in Box 8-1.

Box 8-1

Taking a Patient's Blood Pressure

To manually take a patient's blood pressure, you should follow these steps:

- Have the patient sit down comfortably in a chair, feet flat on the ground and arms on the seat rests, for 10-15 minutes. Ask if he or she has been physically active, has experienced stress, or has eaten or consumed any caffeinated products in the 30 minutes prior. Also ask if the patient has had any new medications or significant changes in his or her medication regimen.

- Decide whether the person needs a regular (majority of patients) or large cuff.

- Locate the brachial artery on the inner upper arm.

continued on page 58

Box 8-1

continued from page 57

- Wrap the cuff around the upper arm with the lower edge positioned one inch from the bend of the inner elbow. Make sure that the cuff is snug, but not tight. (As a guide, you should be able to slip two fingers underneath the cuff.)

- Position the manometer at eye level.

- Position the stethoscope bell comfortably alongside the brachial artery and begin to inflate the cuff. Cease inflation when you no longer hear a pulse through the stethoscope.

- Slowly release the cuff no faster than 2-3 mm/Hg/sec by watching the manometer.

- The first clear sound (similar to a heart beat) you will hear defines the systolic blood pressure (SBP). The last clear audible sound will be the patient's diastolic blood pressure.

- Rapidly deflate the cuff after you have recorded both readings.

- Wait approximately 5 minutes before repeating the procedure.

TABLE 8-4. Blood Pressure (BP) Ranges and Hypertension (HTN)

Blood pressure (BP)	Classification
<120/80	Optimal
SBP 120-139 or DBP 80-89	Prehypertensive
SBP 140-159 or DBP 90-99	HTN, Stage I
SBP ≥160 or DBP ≥100	HTN, Stage II

Note: SBP = systolic blood pressure; DBP = diastolic blood pressure

Pain

Pain is the most difficult vital sign to determine in a patient because its quantitative value is entirely dependent on the patient's perception and lack of comfort. However, being able to assess a patient's pain is crucial because multiple studies have shown that individuals with untreated pain tend to have a poorer outcome and a decreased quality of life.

The classic pain scale ranges from 0 (no pain) to 10 (worst pain imaginable). In addition to asking a patient where on the scale he or she would classify the pain, it is also important to ask some very important follow-up questions, which are listed in Box 8-2.

Box 8-2

Questions About Pain

After asking patients how they would rate their pain on a scale of 1 to 10, follow up with these questions.

1. Is the pain better, the same, or worse?

continued on page 60

Box 8-2

continued from page 59

2. Does the pain remain localized in the same region or is it diffuse?

3. Is the pain relieved with your current drug regimen?

4. Does your pain become worse with movement?

5. Have you had this sort of pain before in your life?

Notes

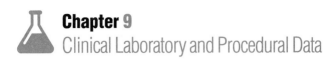

Chapter 9
Clinical Laboratory and Procedural Data

There are a multitude of clinical laboratory tests and diagnostic procedures available for clinicians. The tables in this chapter identify and describe some of these key procedures.

TABLE 9-1. Medical Procedures and Diagnostics

Diagnostic Procedure	Site of Examination	Description
Amniocentesis	Fluid from the sac surrounding the fetus	Fetal abnormalities
Angiography	Any artery in the body	X-ray study in which dye is used to detect a blockage or defect of an artery
Auscultation	Heart	Listening with a stethoscope for abnormal heart and breath sounds
Barium X-ray studies	Gastrointestinal (i.e., esophagus, stomach)	X-ray study to detect ulcers, tumors, or other GI abnormalities
Biopsy	Any tissue in the body	Removal and examination of tissue sample under a microscope for cancer or abnormalities
Bone marrow aspiration	Hipbone or breastbone	Bone marrow sample examined under a microscope for abnormalities
Bronchoscopy	Airways of the lungs	Direct examination for a tumor or other abnormality
Cardiac catheterization	Heart	Study of heart function and structure

continued on page 62

TABLE 9-1. *continued*

Diagnostic Procedure	Site of Examination	Description
Catheter	Heart and/or blood vessels	Tubular instrument passed through blood vessels for vascular and cardiac imaging, diagnosis, and treatment
Colonoscopy	Large intestine	Direct examination for a tumor or other abnormality
Colposcopy	Cervix	Direct examination of the cervix
Computed tomography (CT)	Any part of the body	Computer-enhanced X-ray study to detect structural abnormalities
Culture (Cx)	Sample from any area of the body	Examination of microorganisms grown from a sample to identify infection
Digital rectal exam (DRE)	Inner rectum and prostate	Examination of the prostate to help determine abnormal enlarging
Dual X-ray absorptiometry (DEXA)	Bones (i.e., hip, spine)	Study of bone mineral content using a type of X-ray
Echocardiography (ECHO)	Heart	Study of heart structure and function using sound waves
Electrocardiography (ECG)	Heart	Study of the heart's electrical activity
Electroencephalography (EEG)	Brain	Study of brain's electrical function
Electromyography	Muscles	Recording of a muscle's electrical activity
Endoscopic retrograde cholangiopancreatography (ERCP)	Biliary tract	X-ray study of the biliary tract after injection of a dye
Endoscopy	Digestive tract	Direct examination of internal structures using a flexible viewing tube passed through the mouth

continued on page 63

TABLE 9-1. *continued*

Diagnostic Procedure	Site of Examination	Description
Enzyme-linked immunosorbent assay (ELISA)	Blood and other bodily fluids	The sample is mixed with allergens or microorganisms to test for presence of specific antibodies
Fluoroscopy	Digestive tract, heart, lungs	A continuous X-ray study that allows a doctor to see the inside of an organ as it functions
Intravenous urography	Kidneys, urinary tract	X-ray study of the kidneys and urinary tract after intravenous injection of a dye
Joint aspiration	Joints between bones (i.e., hips, knees)	Examination of fluid from the space within joints for blood cells, crystals, and organisms
Laparoscopy	Abdomen	Direct examination for diagnosis and treatment of abnormalities in the abdomen
Magnetic resonance imaging (MRI)	Any part of the body	Magnetic imaging test for any structural abnormality
Mammography	Breasts	X-ray study for breast cancer
Occult blood test	Large intestine	Test to detect blood in the stool
Papanicolaou test (Pap)	Cervix	Examination under a microscope of cells scraped from the cervix to detect cancer
Paracentesis	Abdomen	Insertion of a needle into the abdominal cavity to remove fluid for examination
Percutaneous transhepatic cholangiography (PTHC)	Liver, biliary tract	X-ray study of the liver and biliary system after dye injection into an intrahepatic bile duct

continued on page 64

TABLE 9-1. *continued*

Diagnostic Procedure	Site of Examination	Description
Positron emission tomography (PET)	Brain and heart	Radioactive imaging to detect abnormality of function
Pulmonary function tests (PFT)	Lungs	Assesses the lungs' capacity to properly respirate and to exchange oxygen and carbon dioxide
Radionuclide imaging	Many organs	Radioactive imaging to detect abnormalities of blood flow, structure, or function
Retrograde urography	Bladder, ureters	X-ray study of the bladder and ureters after infusion of a dye
Sigmoidoscopy	Rectum and last portion of the large intestine	Direct examination to detect tumors or other abnormalities
Spinal tap (lumbar puncture)	Spinal canal	Test for abnormalities of spinal fluid, especially infections
Spirometry	Lungs	Test of lung function that involves blowing into a measuring device
Stress test (exercise tolerance)	Heart	Test of heart function with exertion
Thoracentesis	Space surrounding lungs (pleura)	Removal of fluid from the chest with a needle to detect abnormalities
Thoracoscopy	Lungs	Examination of the pleural space through a viewing tube
Ultrasonography (ultrasound scanning)	Any part of the body	Ultrasound imaging to detect structural or functional abnormalities
Urinalysis	Kidneys and urinary tract	Chemical analysis of urine sample to detect protein, sugar, ketones, and blood cells

TABLE 9-2. Laboratory Values For Blood, Serum, or Fluid Analysis

Blood, Serum or Fluid	Normal Result
α-fetoprotein	Adult: <15 ng/mL
Ammonia (NH_3)	20-70 µg/dL
Ammonia Nitrogen	15-45 µg/dL
Amylase	35-118 IU/L
Bicarbonate: Arterial	21-28 mEq/L
Bilirubin: Conjugated (direct)	≤0.2 mg/dL
Bilirubin: Total	0.1-1 mg/dL
Calcium: Total	8.6-10.3 mg/dL
Calcium: Ionized	4.4-5.1 mg/dL
Chloride	95-110 mEq/L
Prothrombin time (PT)	10-13 sec
Creatinine	0.5-1.7 mg/dL
Glucose, fasting	65-115 mg/dL
Fibrinogen	200-400 mg/dL
Hematocrit (Hct), female	36%-44.6%
Hematocrit (Hct), male	40.7%-50.3%
Hgb_{A1C}	5.3%-7.5% of total Hgb
Hemoglobin (Hgb), female	12.1-15.3 g/dL
Hemoglobin (Hgb), male	13.8-17.5 g/dL
WBC	$3.8-10.0 \times 10^3/\mu L$
RBC, female	$3.5-5 \times 10^6/\mu L$
RBC, male	$4.3-5.9 \times 10^6/\mu L$
Neutrophils	$3.0-7.0 \times 10^6/\mu L$
Mean corpuscular volume (MCV)	80-97.6 µm³
Mean corpuscular hemoglobin (MCH)	27-33 pg/cell
Mean corpuscular hemoglobin concentrate (MCHC)	33-36 g/dL
Erythrocyte sedimentation rate (ESR)	≤20 mm/hr (increases with age)
Glucose-6-phosphate dehydrogenase (G6PD)	$250-5000$ units/10^6 cells
Ferritin	10-383 ng/mL
Folic acid (serum)	2–20 µg/mL
Folate (red blood cell)	140–628 µg/mL
Platelet count	$140-400 \times 10^3/L$
Reticulocytes	0.5%-1.5% of erythrocytes
Vitamin B_{12}	223-1132 pg/mL
Iron, female	30-160 µg/dL
Iron, male	45-160 µg/dL
Iron binding capacity	220-420 µg/dL

continued on page 66

TABLE 9-2. *continued*

Blood, Serum or Fluid	Normal Result
Lactate dehydrogenase (LDH)	
Venous	0.5–2.2 mEq/L
Arterial	0.5–1.6 mEq/L
Lactic acid (lactate)	6-19 mg/dL
Lipase	10-150 units/L
Total Cholesterol	
Desirable	<200 mg/dL
Borderline-high	200-239 mg/dL
High	>239 mg/dL
LDL (goal)	<100 mg/dL
LDL (optimal)	<70 mg/dL
HDL	
Low	<40 mg/dL
Desirable	≥60 mg/dL
Triglycerides	
Desirable	<150 mg/dL
Borderline-high	150-199 mg/dL
High	200-499 mg/dL
Very high	≥500 mg/dL
Magnesium	1.3-2.2 mEq/L
Osmolality	280-300 mOsm/kg
Oxygen saturation (arterial)	94%-100%
pCO_2, arterial	35-45 mm Hg
pH, arterial	7.35-7.45
Phosphorus, inorganic (phosphate)	2.5-4.5 mg/dL
Potassium	3.5-5 mEq/L
Prolactin	0–23 µg/L (increased if pregnant)
Prostate specific antigen (PSA)	0-4 µg/mL
Albumin	3.2-5 g/dL
Rheumatoid factor (RF)	0–20 IU/mL
Sodium	135-147 mEq/L
Thyroid-stimulating hormone (TSH)	0.35-6.2 µU/mL
Thyroxine-binding globulin capacity	10-26 µg/dL
Total triiodothyronine (T3)	80-200 ng/dL
Total thyroxine by RIA (T4)	4-11 µg/dL
AST (aspartate aminotransferase)	11-47 IU/L
ALT (alanine aminotransferase)	7-53 IU/L
Transferrin	220-425 mg/dL (lower in pediatrics and newborns)

continued on page 67

TABLE 9-2. *continued*

Blood, Serum or Fluid	Normal Result
Urea nitrogen (BUN)	8-25 mg/dL
Uric acid, male	3.4–7.0 mg/dL
Uric acid, female	2.4–6.0 mg/dL
Vitamin A (retinol)	15-60 µg/dL
Zinc	50-150 µg/dL

TABLE 9-3. Urinalysis Laboratory Values

Urine Sample	Normal Result
Catecholamines (24hr)	<110 µg
Creatinine, child	8-22 mg/kg
Creatinine, adolescent	8-30 mg/kg
Creatinine, female	11-20 mg/kg
Creatinine, male	14-26 mg/kg
Glucose (24hr)	<0.5 g/day
pH	4.5-8
Protein	1-14 mg/dL
Specific gravity (SG)	1.002-1.030
Uric acid (24hr)	250-750 mg

Sources

Fishbach, F. *A Manual of Laboratory and Diagnostic Tests.* 7th ed. Philadelphia, PA: Lippincott Williams & Wilkins; 2004.

Grundy SM, Cleeman JI, Merz CN, et al. Implications of Recent Clinical Trials for the National Cholesterol Education Program Adult Treatment Panel III Guidelines. *J Am Coll Cardiol.* 2004;44(3):720-32.

Notes

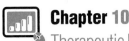

One of the most basic and constant responsibilities of a pharmacist is to monitor a patient's current medication regimen for appropriateness and make or suggest necessary adjustments. Therapeutic drug monitoring (TDM) helps show a relationship between plasma drug concentration and desired clinical or adverse effects.

> TDM helps show a relationship between plasma drug concentration and desired clinical or adverse effects.

TDM and OTC Medications

Very few, if any, over-the-counter (OTC) medications need TDM and modification. This explains why OTC drugs are allowed to be marketed and sold to the general public without a prescription.

However, that is not to imply that OTC drugs should not be monitored and modified in certain circumstances. During your PPEs you may encounter patients and situations in which you judge TDM to be necessary. See Box 10-1 for an example.

Box 10-1

When TDM is Needed

Below are two possible situations you might encounter with your patients.

Patient Situation 1
PT is a 24-year-old male who is complaining of shoulder

continued on page 70

Box 10-1

continued from page 69

pain after taking part in an intramural football game. He has no significant past medical history and is not taking any medications. Per his parent's advice, he wants to take 325 mg of aspirin to help relieve the pain.

Patient Situation 2

JW is an 85-year-old female with a history of bleeding abnormalities who is not currently stabilized on warfarin (INR 2-3) for PE prophylaxis. She is complaining of generalized aches and pains along with a mild headache and wants to take 325 mg of aspirin as her friend instructed her.

In these examples, both patients are seeking the same OTC medication, aspirin, but have very different medical histories that a pharmacist must take into account when deciding what to recommend. An otherwise healthy individual, such as PT, can usually tolerate aspirin well, so it is an appropriate choice to treat his pain. However, for the elderly patient JW, who has bleeding issues, is taking multiple medications, and presents a host of potential co-morbidities, risks versus benefits must be assessed when you consider possible treatments.

However, it would not be prudent to immediately dismiss the use of aspirin in this elderly patient. Instead, a thorough review of her medical history and medications should be done to determine if she can, in fact, be given aspirin while being closely monitored.

The Value of TDM

For some medications, TDM is essential. For example, when a patient is taking phenytoin, which has non-linear or atypical pharmacokinetic components, a small change in dose can result in a significant response. In such cases, TDM is necessary in order to assess safety and efficacy in the patient and prevent adverse effects. TDM is also effective to determine whether a peak or trough concentration is efficacious or toxic in a particular patient (see Box 10-2).

Box 10-2

TDM and Peak or Trough Concentration

The situation below demonstrates how a simple and appropriately drawn level can help determine whether a patient is experiencing adverse events that are associated with a medication.

Patient Situation

LM, a patient with epilepsy, was experiencing abdominal pain. The pharmacist obtained an appropriately drawn trough concentration, and it was determined to be 180 µg/ml. Valproic acid (syrup) has a therapeutic range of 50-100 µg/ml for the treatment of epilepsy. This elevated concentration may suggest that the patient is experiencing an adverse event associated with a too-high dose, or that some other mitigating factor exists.

Prior to incorporating and utilizing TDM, the process of selecting a medication regimen for a patient includes multiple variables that must be taken into account. The responsibility to collect these data should be shared among the entire medical team including physicians, pharmacists, and nurses.

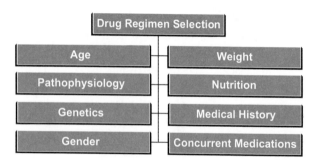

Figure 10-1. Selecting a Drug Regimen.

As illustrated in Figure 10-1, dealing with multiple patient issues necessitates a multidisciplinary approach to not only monitoring medications, but to selecting the initial regimen as well.

Components of TDM

To begin the process of TDM, one must first understand its components.

Therapeutic Range

The therapeutic range, an approximation of the average plasma drug concentration (Table 10-1), describes the dosage range that is safe and efficacious in most patients. These values are derived from patient studies. Due to the multi-factorial issues associated with drug monitoring and patient care, the therapeutic range is never an absolute value.

Steady State (C_{ss})

Steady state is described as the rate of drug administration equaling the rate of drug elimination. In its simplest form, it represents "how much goes in = how much goes out." In most cases, it is attained after 4-5 half-lives ($t_{1/2}$) and there are certain assumptions you can make when analyzing it:

- Dose regimen is not altered.

- Clearance is not altered.

TABLE 10-1. Examples of Medications and Their Therapeutic Ranges

Drug	Range
Valproic acid	50-125 µg/mL
Lithium	0.6-1.2 mEq/L
Lidocaine	2-5 mg/L
Phenytoin	10-20 µg/mL

As successive doses are administered to a patient, the drug begins to accumulate in the body. At a certain point in therapy, the amount of drug administered during a dosing interval equals the amount of drug excreted. When this equilibrium occurs, the peak [P] and trough [T] drug concentrations are the same for each additional dose given. When [P] and [T] are the same with two or more successive doses, C_{ss} is reached.

As with many pharmacokinetic analyses, it is important to realize how certain deviations in administration or other properties would affect steady state:

- Size of a dose does not alter the number of $t_{1/2}$'s it takes to get to C_{ss}.

- Length of $t_{1/2}$ does not alter the number of $t_{1/2}$'s it takes to get to C_{ss}.

- Dosage regimen (pulse dosing vs. continuous infusion) does not alter the number of $t_{1/2}$'s it takes to get to C_{ss}.

Therapeutic ranges provide important information for medication monitoring. However, also keep in mind that you are always treating the patient, not just the numbers.

Steps in Drug Monitoring

Drug monitoring is a multi-step process.

Step 1: Decide What the Medication Indication is in a Particular Patient.

Medical care relies on an appropriate diagnosis based on a patient's clinical signs, symptoms, past medical history, concurrent medications, and procedural and laboratory data. Become integrated with the medical team and make sure that you provide input on the differential and final diagnosis in each patient. Analyzing the patient's current or recent medications—a role that is ideal for a pharmacist—can help the team identify a good percentage of disease states.

Step 2: Assess the Need for Serum Drug Concentrations and Monitoring.

Not all drugs administered to patients need therapeutic monitoring. Needlessly ordering levels when they will shed little information on efficacy or safety in a patient can waste hospital resources, incur unnecessary patient charges, and in the case of critical patients and pediatric patients, cause dramatic changes in blood loss.

Step 3: Decide What Therapeutic Range is Appropriate for this Patient and Assess the Need for a Loading Dose.

A drug does not necessarily have the same range of therapeutic levels for different indications. Furthermore, a medication that is being used acutely versus chronically may have entirely different therapeutic ranges. Finally, some indications require a titration, which can make it more difficult to interpret a level until the upper limits of titration are reached in the patient's regimen.

Step 4: Verify Whether the Drug Concentration is Truly a Peak or Trough.

Multiple factors can cause therapeutic range deviations (see Table 10-2). Make sure you know if the referenced therapeutic range is based on a peak or trough concentration because you cannot successfully do TDM by utilizing incorrect parameters. In addition, verify that the level was drawn at the appropriate time, as stipulated in the literature or product insert. Finally, if the level still seems incorrect or atypical, go back to the medication administration record (MAR) and confirm that the correct dose of the medication was administered at the correct time.

Equations to Help With TDM

Various pharmacokinetic equations exist to assist pharmacists with TDM. Several of them are illustrated below.

Volume of Distribution (V_D)

Volume of distribution refers to the apparent volume required to account for all of the drug in the body's tissues (i.e., heart, bone, brain) and can be useful in calculating loading doses and determining the expected peak serum concentration (see Figure 10-2). However, the V_D by itself will not help calculate maintenance doses for patients.

TABLE 10-2. Possible Causes of Therapeutic Range Deviations

Lower than anticipated	Higher than anticipated	Within range, but patient not responding clinically
• Patient compliance	• Patient compliance	• Tolerance (receptor)
• Drug regimen error	• Drug regimen error	• Drug regimen error
• Formulation error (extended release vs. immediate release)	• Formulation error (extended release vs. immediate release)	• Renal and/or hepatic function issues
• Poor bioavailability	• High bioavailability	• Drug interaction
• Rapid elimination	• Slow elimination	• Co-morbidities
• ↓ plasma protein binding	• ↑ plasma protein binding	
• C_{ss} not reached	• Blood sample timing	
• Blood sample timing	• Renal and/or hepatic function issues	
• Renal and/or hepatic function issues	• Drug interaction (enzyme inhibitors)	
• Drug interaction (enzyme inducers)		

Load (dose) ⟶ $$\frac{LD}{V_d} = \Delta C_p$$ ⟵ Peak Serum Concentration
Volume of Distribution

Figure 10-2. V_D Shown in an Equation for Determining Loading Doses and Peak Serum Concentration.

Clearance (Cl)

Clearance refers to the blood volume which is fully cleared of a drug in a given time period (see Figure 10-3), assuming linear behavior. This parameter can assist in calculating maintenance doses in order to achieve a desired C_{ss}, but Cl by itself will not help determine a loading dose.

Dosage Rate $\longrightarrow$ $\dfrac{DR}{Cl} = C_{ss}$ $\longleftarrow$ Steady State

Clearance $\longrightarrow$

Figure 10-3. Clearance Shown in an Equation for Determining Dosage.

Other useful TDM equations and parameters include those found in Figures 10-4, 10-5, 10-6, and 10-7.

Clearance $\longrightarrow$ $\dfrac{Cl}{V_D} = k_e$ $\longleftarrow$ Elimination Rate Constant

Volume of Distribution $\longrightarrow$

Figure 10-4. Elimination Rate Constant.

$$\frac{0.693}{k_e} = \frac{0.693(V_D)}{Cl} = t_{1/2}$$

Figure 10-5. Determination of Half-Life ($t_{1/2}$).

$$\frac{\ln(C1/C2)}{k_e} = t_{1/2}$$

Figure 10-6. Determination of Half-Life ($t_{1/2}$) Using Two Concentrations.

$$\frac{K_o(1 - e^{-Kt})e^{-KT}}{V_D \cdot K(1 - e^{-K})} = C_{ssp}$$

Figure 10-7. Calculation of Peak Steady State Concentration Using Multiple Parameters.

Notes

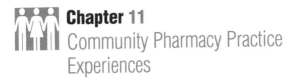

Chapter 11
Community Pharmacy Practice Experiences

The majority of pharmacy candidates will have some experience in community retail pharmacies through workshops, internships, or part-time employment. Under the supervision of an affiliated faculty preceptor from the pharmacy school, you will practice skills essential for the effective delivery of patient care.

If you are not placed in an independently owned retail pharmacy, you will probably be assigned to one of the major pharmacy chains (see Table 11-1).

> The majority of pharmacy candidates will have some experience in community retail pharmacies.

Table 11-1. Some Well-Known Chain Pharmacies in the United States

Name
• Walgreens
• CVS
• Target
• Wal-Mart
• Longs Drugs
• Rite Aid

If you have already worked in any one of these pharmacies, it is likely you will be assigned to a different chain. Some may argue that it is best to remain where you already know the protocols, system, and workflow. However, being exposed to an entirely dissimilar way of approaching dispensing, counseling, record-keeping, and prescription entry during your PPE will diversify your training and help you learn different ways of approaching tasks.

Interacting With Your Colleagues

It is important for you to interact positively with your colleagues in the community pharmacy. In addition to working with your pharmacist preceptor (usually the pharmacy manager or a staff pharmacist) you will develop working relationships with the pharmacy technicians and possibly even employees outside of the pharmacy, such as the store manager, floor clerks, etc. Some community retail PPEs may also provide exposure to corporate aspects of the operation and give you the opportunity to meet executive and upper level administration, such as regional pharmacy managers and the Director of Operations.

Special Projects During Community PPEs

During your PPE, you may take part in many projects in the pharmacy and also in outreach efforts in the community. These may include:

- "Brown-bag" lunches for store staff and community members to educate them about their current medications.

- In-services for the pharmacy on workflow and process improvements.

- Disease state informational sessions for staff and community.

- Antibiotic follow-up for adults and children.

Community Pharmacy Tasks

In addition to these projects and opportunities, there are some basic skills that you will be required to demonstrate. Practicing the following tasks will sharpen your retail pharmacy and patient care skills.

Tasks you may be asked to perform include:

- Entering a patient prescription at the receiving window and/or by fax, email, and telephone.

- Starting and/or updating a patient's medication profile.

- Checking a patient's allergies and noting the specific type of reaction(s).

- Submitting a prescription insurance claim electronically or manually.

- Filling a prescription and applying the correct label to the vial.

- Verifying the finished product against the original prescription order.

- Counseling the patient upon receiving the prescription, especially if it is for a new medication.

- Filling prescriptions appropriately according to the pharmacy's standard practice.

- Working on inventory control, including controlled substances (CV-CII).

- Managing the employee schedule.

- Counseling for and recommending OTC products.

- Contacting third party insurers for issues relating to a patient's medication coverage.

- Discussing any prior authorization problems with the patient, health care professional and/or state health department.

Since you are considered a temporary employee at your retail pharmacy, you must abide by that specific company's rules and regulations, including those covering dress code, breaks/lunch schedules, and patient interaction. Make sure that you go over these specific company policies with preceptors or the store manager. Even something as simple as parking improperly could lead to unnecessary complications during your PPE.

Notes

Chapter 12
Hospital Pharmacy Practice Experiences

The hospital is the second most common setting in which you or your colleagues may work during PPEs. Your placement will be in a private or state-run institution, which may or may not be affiliated with a university or college.

> In this PPE setting, you may work as a pharmacy technician or in another hospital department.

In this PPE setting, you may work as a pharmacy technician or in another hospital department. Your duties will usually focus on the medical center's inpatient pharmacy dispensing services. Having access to complete patient records and histories will allow you to develop the most complete and accurate medication regimens. You may also have the opportunity to witness and/or participate in clinical services, although this is not your primary responsibility.

Special Projects During Hospital PPEs

There are several types of intensive projects that hospital preceptors may require you to complete. The most common are Journal Clubs, Drug Monographs, and Patient Cases.

Journal Club
Select one peer-reviewed journal article pertinent to the practice of inpatient dispensing or another suitable topic. Determine who will be your audience and whether or not the presentation should be done in a formal or informal manner. Furthermore, because you will have a hectic schedule in the hospital inpatient setting, make sure you allow enough time to complete your journal club.

Drug Monograph

A monograph, one of the most difficult projects you will be assigned during your PPE, requires the author to write extensively about all aspects of a particular medication and compare it to another medication in the same class (or a competitor). Often the monograph will be set up and answered so the student or preceptor can present findings to a P&T Committee for formulary inclusion or exclusion.

The difficult aspect of this project is to make sure that your monograph is your original work and not just a copy of a particular medication's package insert (which could be interpreted as plagiarism and lead to possible disciplinary action). To avoid just copying material directly from a package insert, utilize the following suggestions.

- Read over the package to get a firm understanding of the drug and its properties.

- Do a literature search and find review articles pertaining to your medication or the original research studies used for the drug's approval.

- Utilize the package insert for certain sections that cannot be changed or worded very differently, such as pharmacokinetics, and cite the insert as a reference.

When comparing your drug to a competitor or established formulary medication, you should include, at a minimum, two well designed clinical trials (randomized, double-blind, placebo controlled investigations). Do not forget to include your own critical analysis of not only the competitor drug, but also your own chosen medication to provide an unbiased recommendation.

Patient Case

The patient case can be seen as the culmination of your PPE. Although you are working in the central pharmacy and providing dispensing services, you still have access to enough patient information to create a successful and detailed case. Incorporate as much data as you can to make your patient case as specific, accurate, and complete as possible.

Hospital Pharmacy Tasks

There are a number of skills that you will utilize and perfect while at the medical center. They include:

- Entering a patient order primarily through fax, electronically, and by telephone.

- Modifying an inpatient medication profile.

- Checking a patient's allergies and noting the specific types of reactions.

- Noting in the patient progress note any significant disease states that may interfere with a medication regimen.

- Filling a prescription and applying the correct labeling to the container.

- Assisting in the preparation of unit dose medications for patient use.

- Verifying the finished product against the original prescription order.

- Filling prescriptions appropriately according to the pharmacy's standard practice.

- Doing inventory control, including controlled substances (CV-CII).

- Managing the employee schedule.

- Contacting physicians, nurses, and clinical pharmacists for any irregularities or abnormalities in a patient's medication regimen.

- Assisting the hospital staff with formulary issues regarding specific medications.

- Discussing medication safety and adverse event reporting.

- Preparing and dispensing IV products in a clean sterile environment.

- Working with hazardous materials and medications such as compounding components and chemotherapeutic drugs.

- Replenishing the hospital's crash carts consistently.

Notes

Chapter 13
Chronic/Long-Term-Care Pharmacy Practice Experiences

Life expectancy is increasing as medical technology and drug breakthroughs combat diseases more effectively. As a result, the number of long-term-care (LTC) facilities, such as nursing centers and rehabilitation homes for the elderly, is increasing, meaning there is a greater need for monitoring of patients' conditions and progress. This role traditionally falls to the LTC consultant pharmacist, who is in charge of monitoring, evaluating, and recommending therapeutic changes in these facilities and homes. The consultant pharmacist will usually serve as your preceptor during your LTC PPE.

> The LTC consultant pharmacist will usually serve as your preceptor during your PPE.

The majority of LTC facilities are owned and managed by a central corporation or firm. This corporation may have an affiliated pharmacy or contract for services with an outside pharmacy. LTC pharmacies may provide dispensing services, pharmacist consultations, or both.

What's Different About the LTC Pharmacy
There are particular characteristics of this type of PPE that distinguish it from others. These considerations will affect how you assess your patients' medications and make recommendations.

Visits to Different Facilities
Consultant pharmacists may travel to an LTC only a few times a month. If the LTC is managed by a large company that has

numerous facilities, a pharmacist may visit each location only once per month. Working in different LTC locations during your PPE will allow you to see how different facilities, even those owned by the same company, practice patient care.

Busy Physicians and Pharmacists

There may only be one or two physicians assigned to a particular facility. These physicians may also have multiple other facility assignments, in addition to duties at a hospital or private practice. LTC pharmacists often have responsibility for a large number of patients; a consultant pharmacist may review up to 200 charts in a single day for patients on multiple medications. The demands of the LTC setting mean you must be aware of the potential for confusion and errors.

Regulations for Laboratory Work

Laboratory draws are often very tightly regulated in the LTC sector due to costs, convenience, and reimbursement issues. Although drugs such as anticoagulants and neurologic medications usually require tight monitoring and frequent assessment, LTC facilities and their protocols will often stipulate how many times blood draws are suggested or allowed. Make sure that you pay close attention to these protocols and be aware of how they may impact patient care.

Communicating with Medical Staff

Since LTC physicians often juggle multiple responsibilities, it can be difficult to contact them to discuss a treatment issue or recommendation. Most recommendations and suggestions from the consultant pharmacist are written in the patient's chart or on a message placed in the physician's mailbox, but these notes may not be read until the next time he or she visits the facility. Therefore, make sure that you plan ahead in case your recommendations are not considered right away.

Adhering to Protocols

Practicing pharmacy in the LTC sector requires adapting to state, federal, and individual company protocols. For instance, you are required to make sure patients sign a consent form before you administer many psychiatric medications. Check for this form in the patient's chart; if it is not there, notify your preceptor or the nursing staff.

LTC Pharmacy Tasks

There are a number of tasks and responsibilities that you may be required to complete while on an LTC PPE. They include:

> Practicing pharmacy in the LTC sector requires adapting to state, federal, and individual company protocols.

- Providing in-services to the nursing and support staff.

- Participating in protocol and quality assessments, especially in the area of falls prevention.

- Checking medication rooms for properly stored medications and disposing of expired drugs.

- Maintaining and checking the controlled substance inventory.

- Disposing of unused controlled substances or preparing them for return to the dispensing pharmacy.

- Entering, filling, and dispensing medication at the pharmacy affiliated or owned by the LTC company.

- Presenting a journal club and/or patient case to the pharmacy and administrative staff.

Notes

Chapter 14
Ambulatory/Acute Care Pharmacy Practice Experiences

The need for ambulatory and acute care pharmacists has increased at an astonishing pace. Multiple opportunities are available in these settings to participate directly in patient care and assessment. The majority of ambulatory care clinics are affiliated with a medical center, although stand-alone clinics and those within a retail pharmacy setting are also gaining popularity and market share.

> The advantage of doing a PPE in the ambulatory or acute care setting is that you will utilize clinical skills not normally expected of you in other pharmacy sectors.

The advantage of doing a PPE in the ambulatory or acute care setting is that you will utilize clinical skills not normally expected of you in other pharmacy sectors (such as supervising a patient's anticoagulation therapy, initiating a smoking cessation plan, or determining a proper oral contraceptive) and also obtain in-depth disease state and therapeutic knowledge.

Keep in mind that in the ambulatory or acute care setting, you may only see each patient a few times during your PPE. Therefore, it is important to utilize your time with patients to gather as much information as possible. As in the LTC PPE, plan your pharmaceutical care based on a long-term approach, since the patient may not return to the clinic for a month.

Ambulatory/Acute Care PPE Tasks and Specialty Clinics

Within this sector, there are a wide variety of opportunities for you. You may be assigned to different types of clinics that require their own pharmacy skills sets and clinical practice parameters (see Table 14-1).

Prior to beginning at a particular site, or during the first few days, familiarize yourself with any point of care (POC) devices, such as those testing blood glucose, cholesterol, and bone density.

TABLE 14-1. Ambulatory Care Specialty Sites and Possible PPE Responsibilities

Clinic	Description	Roles and Responsibilities
Amiodarone	Patients who are on amiodarone for an established indication (usually arrhythmia)	Medication dosing, monitoring, and modification
Anticoagulation	Patients who need anticoagulation secondary to procedures or increased risk per medical history	Medication dosing, monitoring, and modification; POC INR/PT testing
Diabetes	Diabetic patients who need assistance in assessing their diabetic control and progression	Medication dosing, monitoring, and modification; POC glucose & Hgb_{AIC} testing; device counseling
Dialysis	Patients undergoing dialysis and in need of medication assessment	Medication dosing, monitoring, and modification

continued on page 93

TABLE 14-1. *continued*

Clinic	Description	Roles and Responsibilities
Family Medicine	Adults and children with a wide range of medical issues	Medication dosing, monitoring, and modification; physical exam; vaccinations; device counseling; insurance and third-party claims; patient assistance program enrollment
Geriatrics	Elderly patients with multiple medical problems and extensive medication regimens	Medication dosing, monitoring, and modification
GI	Patients with a GI-related disease state	Medication dosing, monitoring, and modification
Heart Failure	Patients who are diagnosed with heart failure	Medication dosing, monitoring, and modification; quality of life assessment
ID/HIV	Patients who need follow-up for an infectious process or who have been diagnosed with HIV/AIDS	Medication dosing, monitoring, and modification; administration technique
Medication Therapy Management (MTM)	Patients with extensive number of medications	Medication dosing, monitoring, and modification; insurance and third-party claims; patient assistance program enrollment
Neurology	Post-surgical patients or those with neuro-logical pathologies or processes	Medication dosing, monitoring, and modification
Oncology	Patients undergoing chemotherapy for treatment of tumors	Medication dosing, monitoring, and modification

continued on page 94

TABLE 14-1. *continued*

Clinic	Description	Roles and Responsibilities
Pain	Patients experiencing chronic pain	Medication dosing, monitoring, and modification; equianalgesic conversions
Pediatrics	Those patients <19 years of age with various medical issues	Medication dosing, monitoring, and modification; height, weight and nutritional assessment
Psychiatry	Patients diagnosed with psychiatric illnesses or mental deficits	Medication dosing, monitoring, and modification
Pulmonary & Asthma	Patients who have chronic pulmonary issues (i.e., asthma, emphysema)	Medication dosing, monitoring, and modification; spirometry; device technique (inhalers); asthma action plans
Smoking Cessation	Patients interested in quitting smoking	Medication dosing, monitoring, and modification; smoking cessation diary/log
Transplant	Patients who have undergone a solid organ transplant	Medication dosing, monitoring, and modification; culture follow-up
Women's Health	Issues pertaining to gynecology and obstetrics, including sexually transmitted diseases	Medication dosing, monitoring, and modification; initiation of birth control and counseling; emergency contraception; infertility assessment

Chapter 15
Advanced Clinical Pharmacy Practice Experiences

One of the most intensive experiences you will undergo during your candidacy is completing one or more Advanced Clinical PPEs. During this time, you will focus on a specific inpatient medical service.

Types of Advanced Clinical PPEs

There are a number of clinical service opportunities available to you in this type of PPE. Some of them are described in the following section, along with duties and experiences typical of each PPE setting.

Surgical Intensive Care Unit (SICU)

This PPE involves providing pharmaceutical care for patients specifically in the SICU, which is generally reserved for critically ill, surgical, and trauma patients. The environment in the SICU is extremely fluid due to patients' unstable conditions.

Your responsibilities in the SICU may include:

- Patient profile review and updating (i.e., allergy information and latest medication list prior to admission).

- Assisting other members of the team with medication order entry and order clarification.

- Daily or twice-daily rounding with the team and support professionals.

- Pharmacokinetic support and recommendations.

- Nutritional support in tandem with dieticians/nutritionists.

- Professional interaction with physicians, nurses, therapists, rehabilitation service, students, and support specialists.

- Participation in grand rounds and/or lecture series.

Areas of Interest in the SICU PPE
Areas of interest commonly associated with this PPE include post-operative infections, DVT prophylaxis, GI stress ulcer prophylaxis, pain control, sedation, monitoring of hemodynamics, sepsis and inflammatory response syndrome (SIRS), nutritional support, pharmacokinetics in critically ill patients, organ failure, fluid replacement, and rehabilitation.

Medical Intensive Care Unit (MICU)
This PPE involves providing pharmaceutical care for those patients in the MICU, which is for critically ill medical patients. Similar to the SICU, the environment in the MICU is in constant flux.

Your responsibilities in the MICU may include:

- Patient profile review and updating (i.e., allergy information and latest medication list prior to admission).

- Assisting other members of the team with medication order entry and order clarification.

- Daily or twice-daily rounding with the team and support professionals.

- Pharmacokinetic support and recommendations.

- Nutritional support in tandem with dieticians/nutritionists.

- Professional interaction with physicians, nurses, therapists, rehabilitation service, students, and support specialists.

- Participation in grand rounds and/or lecture series.

Areas of Interest in the MICU PPE

Areas of interest commonly associated with this PPE include acute respiratory distress syndrome (ARDS), mechanical ventilation, DVT prophylaxis, GI stress ulcer prophylaxis, analgesia, sedation, hemodynamics, sepsis and inflammatory response syndrome (SIRS), nutritional support, pharmacokinetics, multiple organ failure, fluid replacement, acute alcohol withdrawal, DKA, hypertensive emergency/crisis, GI bleeds, status asthmaticus, status epilepticus, overdoses, renal failure, metabolic disturbances, and disseminated intravascular coagulation (DIC).

Pediatric Intensive Care Unit (PICU)

This PPE involves providing pharmaceutical care services to the PICU population. PICU patients range in age from newborns to young adults (up to 18 years of age). This PPE may also provide you with exposure to investigational therapies and studies.

Your responsibilities in the PICU may include:

- Patient profile review and updating (i.e., allergy information and latest medication list prior to admission, if available).

- Assisting other members of the team with medication order entry and order clarification.

- Daily or twice-daily rounding with the team and support professionals.

- Pharmacokinetic support and recommendations.

- Nutritional support in tandem with dieticians/nutritionists.

- Professional interaction with physicians, nurses, therapists, rehabilitation service, students, and support specialists.

- Participation in grand rounds and/or lecture series.

Areas of Interest in the PICU PPE

Areas of interest commonly associated with this PPE include pediatric pharmacotherapy and consequent dosing strategies, post-operative care, sepsis, meningitis, asthma exacerbations (including new onset), status epilepticus, pediatric emergencies, allergies, common infections and cold symptoms, respiratory issues, and nutritional support.

Neonatal Intensive Care Unit (NICU)

This PPE involves providing pharmaceutical care to the NICU patient population. Patients include premature infants (who are usually kept in a separate section of the NICU) to full-term infants with an underlying disease. The NICU experience may expose you to investigational drug studies and new therapies. This PPE can be thought of as a position where pharmacy care is based on "art" and "instinct" versus the textbook, since there can be so many gray areas with this patient population.

Your responsibilities in the NICU may include:

- Patient profile review and updating (i.e., allergy information and latest medication list prior to admission, if available).

- Assisting other members of the team with medication order entry and order clarification.

- Daily or twice-daily rounding with the team and support professionals.

- Pharmacokinetic support and recommendations.

- Nutritional support in tandem with dieticians/nutritionists.

- Professional interaction with physicians, nurses, therapists, rehabilitation service, students, and support specialists.

- Participation in grand rounds and/or lecture series.

Areas of Interest in the NICU PPE

Areas of interest commonly associated with this PPE include neonatal pharmacotherapy and consequent dosing strategies, post-operative care, sepsis, meningitis, asthma exacerbations (including new onset), status epilepticus, pediatric emergencies, allergies, common infections and cold symptoms, multiple and deeply involved respiratory and cardiac issues (i.e., heart defects), and nutritional support.

Transplant Intensive Care Unit (TICU)

This PPE involves providing pharmaceutical care for pre- and post-operative solid organ transplant patients. This service is comprised of health care professionals who perform transplant surgery, supportive care, and LTC for adult and pediatric liver, kidney, and pancreatic recipients. Additionally, patients who develop complications secondary to their transplant are often re-admitted to the TICU for continued care.

Your responsibilities in the TICU may include:

- Intensive patient profile review and updating (i.e., allergy information and latest medication list prior to admission, if available) and recording of proposed immunosuppressive plan (pre- and post-operatively).

- Assisting other members of the team with medication order entry and order clarification.

- Daily or twice-daily rounding with the team and support professionals.

- Pharmacokinetic support and recommendations.

- Nutritional support in tandem with dieticians/nutritionists.

- Professional interaction with physicians, nurses, therapists, rehabilitation service, students, and support specialists.

- Participation in grand rounds and/or lecture series.

Areas of Interest in the TICU PPE

Areas of interest commonly associated with this PPE include surgical techniques of organ transplantation, complications of organ transplantation, immunosuppression, treatment of rejection, nutritional support, pharmacokinetic analysis, and fluids assessment.

Cardiac Intensive Care Unit (CICU)

This PPE involves providing pharmaceutical care for those patients in the CICU and telemetry units. Patients are generally post-operative for cardiac, thoracic, and vascular surgeries and for heart and lung transplants. Additionally, those critical patients with complex cardiac events, such as aneurysms and dissections, may be included in this unit due to the need for intensive monitoring.

Your responsibilities in the CICU may include:

- Patient profile review and updating (i.e., allergy information and latest medication list prior to admission, if available).

- Assisting other members of the team with medication order entry and order clarification.

- Daily or twice-daily rounding with the team and support professionals.

- Pharmacokinetic support and recommendations.

- Nutritional support in tandem with dieticians/nutritionists.

- Professional interaction with physicians, nurses, therapists, rehabilitation service, students, and support specialists.

- Participation in grand rounds and/or lecture series.

Areas of Interest in the CICU PPE

Areas of interest commonly associated with this PPE include post-operative infections, arrhythmias (i.e., atrial fibrillation), GI stress ulcer prophylaxis, analgesia, sedation, hemodynamic monitoring, nutritional support, pharmacokinetics, fluids assessment, post-operative nausea and vomiting (PONV), stents and catheterization, angioplasty, and stress testing.

Neuroscience Intensive Care Unit (Neuro ICU)

This PPE involves providing pharmaceutical care to critically ill patients focusing on neurological events (i.e., surgery and trauma). The Neuro ICU may also include otolaryngology and head and neck patients.

Your responsibilities in the Neuro ICU may include:

- Patient profile review and updating (i.e., allergy information and latest medication list prior to admission, if available).

- Assisting other members of the team with medication order entry and order clarification.

- Daily or twice-daily rounding with the team and support professionals.

- Pharmacokinetic support and recommendations.

- Nutritional support in tandem with dieticians/nutritionists.

- Professional interaction with physicians, nurses, therapists, rehabilitation service, students, and support specialists.

- Participation in grand rounds and/or lecture series.

Areas of Interest in the Neuro ICU PPE

Areas of interest commonly associated with this PPE include post-operative infections, seizures and status epilepticus, GI stress ulcer prophylaxis, analgesia, sedation, EEG monitoring, nutritional support, pharmacokinetics, fluids assessment, post-operative nausea and vomiting (PONV), surgical wound assessments, and neurological deficits and progression.

Infectious Diseases (ID)

This PPE involves being part of an infectious diseases consultation team and possibly working with an affiliated clinic. The team is utilized by any medical service that needs assistance in determining infectious diseases or proper medication regimens and monitoring parameters.

Your responsibilities in an ID PPE may include:

- Patient profile review and updating, especially allergy information.

- Assisting other members of the team with medication order entry and order clarification.

- Daily rounding with the team and support professionals.

- Pharmacokinetic support and recommendations.

- Professional interaction with physicians, nurses, therapists, rehabilitation service, students, and support specialists.

- Designing appropriate antimicrobial therapy regimens.

- Recommending appropriate antimicrobial regimens and monitoring plans.

- Educating patients and medical staff on topics pertaining to infectious diseases.

Areas of Interest in the ID PPE

Areas of interest commonly associated with this PPE include post-operative infections, emerging infectious diseases, bioterrorism, resistance and susceptibility issues, pharmacokinetics, wound assessments, common infections, compliance issues (i.e., HIV/AIDS) and bacterial, viral, and/or fungal culture interpretations.

Hematology and Oncology (HEM-ONC)

This PPE involves providing pharmaceutical care for those patients who are admitted to the hematology and oncology service. Many units will also include patients admitted for a bone marrow transplant.

Your responsibilities during this PPE may include:

- Patient profile review and updating (i.e., allergy information and latest medication list prior to admission, if available).

- Assisting other members of the team with medication order entry and order clarification.

- Daily or twice-daily rounding with the team and support professionals.

- Pharmacokinetic support and recommendations.

- Nutritional support in tandem with dieticians/nutritionists.

- Professional interaction with physicians, nurses, therapists, rehabilitation service, students, and support specialists.

- Participation in grand rounds and/or lecture series.

Areas of Interest in the HEM-ONC Service PPE

Areas of interest commonly associated with this PPE include hematology and oncology disease states, antineoplastic chemotherapy, radiological therapy, investigational drugs, pain management, prophylaxis and treatment of chemotherapy-induced nausea and vomiting, neutropenic fever, hypercalcemia associated with malignancy, toxicities of chemotherapy, and growth-colony stimulating factors (G-CSF).

Gerontology and Geriatrics

This PPE involves providing pharmaceutical care for those patients who are admitted to the gerontology and geriatrics service.

Your responsibilities during this PPE may include:

- Patient profile review and updating (i.e., allergy information and latest medication list prior to admission, if available).

- Assisting other members of the team with medication order entry and order clarification.

- Daily rounding with the team and support professionals.

- Pharmacokinetic support and recommendations.

- Nutritional support in tandem with dieticians/nutritionists.

- Professional interaction with physicians, nurses, therapists, rehabilitation service, students, and support specialists.

- Participation in grand rounds and/or lecture series.

- Coordination with social workers on LTC facility placement or hospice.

- Effective communication with individuals who may have cognitive and/or neurological deficits.

Areas of Interest in the Gerontology and Geriatrics Service PPE

Areas of interest commonly associated with this PPE include physiologic changes that occur as the result of aging, pharmacokinetic and pharmacologic action(s) of medication in this population, angina, bowel and bladder incontinence, anemias, congestive heart failure (CHF), dementias, depression, diabetes, hypertension (HTN), arrhythmias, insomnia, osteoporosis, Parkinson's Disease, pneumonias (community-acquired and hospital-acquired), pressure sores, urinary tract infections (UTI), seizure disorders, bipolar disorder (BPD), and schizophrenia.

Pediatrics

This PPE involves providing pharmaceutical care services to the pediatric patient population. Patients range in age from newborns to young adults (up to 18 years of age). Disease states include general medicine cases and transfers from the PICU and NICU.

Your responsibilities during this PPE may include:

- Patient profile review and updating (i.e., allergy information and latest medication list prior to admission, if available).

- Assisting other members of the team with medication order entry and order clarification.

- Daily or twice-daily rounding with the team and support professionals.

- Pharmacokinetic support and recommendations.

- Nutritional support in tandem with dieticians/nutritionists.

- Professional interaction with physicians, nurses, therapists, rehabilitation service, students and support specialists.

- Participation in grand rounds and/or lecture series.

Areas of Interest in the Pediatric PPE

Areas of interest commonly associated with this PPE include pediatric pharmacotherapy and consequent dosing strategies, post-operative care, sepsis, meningitis, asthma exacerbations (including new onset), status epilepticus, pediatric emergencies, allergies, common infections and cold symptoms, respiratory issues, nutritional support, newly diagnosed diabetics, pediatric chemotherapy, and pediatric emergencies.

Emergency Department (ED) and Toxicology

This PPE involves providing pharmaceutical care services in the ED. This department will serve a hugely varied patient population ranging from newborns to the elderly, who may have extremely traumatic medical issues. Additionally, medication overdoses, both intentional and accidental, will almost always result in the patient first coming to the ED.

Your responsibilities during this PPE may include:

- Initiating and collaborating on a patient profile (i.e., allergy information and medication list prior to admission).

- Assisting other members of the team with medication order entry and order clarification in an acute setting.

- Pharmacokinetic support and recommendations.

- Nutritional support in tandem with dieticians/nutritionists.

- Professional interaction with physicians, nurses, therapists, ambulance officers, rehabilitation service, students, and support specialists.

Areas of Interest in the ED PPE
Areas of interest commonly associated with this PPE include infectious diseases, sexual assaults, emergency contraception, vehicle accidents, gunshots, blunt trauma, burns, overdoses, suicide attempts, sepsis, meningitis, asthma exacerbations (including new onset), status epilepticus, cardiac and/or respiratory arrest, anaphylaxis, common infections and cold symptoms, DKA, hypothermia, alcohol intoxication, withdrawal, toxicology, myocardial infarction, and stroke.

Advanced Clinical PPE Projects
In addition to providing extensive clinical pharmacy coverage during your advanced PPE, you will also be tasked with a good number of projects typical of other PPEs. They include:

- Journal Club

- Drug Monograph

- Patient Case Presentation

- In-Services

- Grand Rounds Presentation

- Committee Participation (as directed by your preceptor)

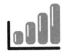

Chapter 16
Business/Management Pharmacy
Practice Experiences

The business sector plays a major role in the practice of pharmacy and offers many career opportunities. As business and management studies become more integrated into the profession, more pharmacy schools are offering PPEs in these areas, in addition to providing business electives during the didactic years.

> Business-oriented PPEs may involve projects ranging from medical writing to clinical trial design and implementation.

Major business entities that may offer PPEs include drug insurance providers and medical writing and consulting firms. Business-oriented PPEs may involve projects ranging from medical writing to clinical trial design and implementation.

In addition, there are also opportunities for PPEs affiliated with drug companies—the largest business sector having a direct effect on the practice of pharmacy and patient care.

Third-Party and Pharmacy Benefit Management (PBM)

Prescription drug insurance providers, often referred to as third parties or PBM, allow individuals to have their prescription drug prices covered depending on which specific plan they are enrolled in. Your role in this process can include formulary management, customer service inquiries, committee meetings, business development, and drug company contract negotiations. In addition, you may also be involved in contacting physicians to suggest a therapeutic alternative to a medication that is either not covered for the patient or is exceptionally expensive.

Insurance Plans

When dealing with drug insurance issues, you should be aware of some of the ways insurance plans work. Some information that may be helpful is listed in Box 16-1.

Box 16-1

Information About Insurance Plans

There are a huge number of prescription drug plans available to consumers, even within one single company.

All plans base their cost on their formulary, which dictates whether a drug is preferred or non-preferred. Preferred drugs will usually be covered to a much higher degree than non-preferred medications, resulting in lower costs to the patient.

Drug plans prefer having patients obtain a prescription for a generically available medication because of cost savings. If a generic is not available, the drug plan may require a prior authorization, where a physician must confirm that the specific medication prescribed is medically necessary.

Medical coverage does not always mean prescription drug coverage. More often than not, individuals may have separate plans for their medical and drug coverage, which should be stated on the patient's identification card or verified by calling the customer service line for the insurance company.

Drug Company PPEs

Medications used to treat disease states are researched, developed, manufactured, and marketed by pharmaceutical companies. Obtaining a PPE at a drug company can be difficult because of the nature of the business, the need for highly experienced professionals, and the company's own regulations dealing with proprietary information. However, if your career goals do include working for the drug industry, it is possible to obtain a PPE position. These companies are definitely aware of the skill sets that pharmacists have to advance drug development, product support, and regulatory affairs, among other areas.

Some aspects of the business that a PPE may cover include:

- Drug and Medical Information

- Product and Pipeline Development

- Sales and Marketing

- Labeling and Medical Writing

- Disease State Background Compilation

- Safety and Adverse Events Analysis

- Clinical Trial Study Analysis

- Quality Control

- Manufacturing Processes

- Formulation Development

- Product Life Cycle Management

- Knowledge Management

- Crisis Control

The Clinical Trial Process

The clinical trial process begins with discovering a new compound, or new molecular entity (NME), during preclinical research and ends with Phase IV post-marketing studies. It is important to note that Phase IV studies never truly conclude, because they are used to continually gather new safety information on reported adverse events.

Preclinical Research

Preclinical research encompasses drug discovery, screening, toxicology, characterization of pharmacology for a compound, and filing of regulatory documentation, specifically an Investigational New Drug (IND) application, for further progression in clinical trials.

Potential compounds can be discovered internally by a company's scientists or acquired from another company.

Phase I

Phase I involves:

- Determination of drug safety and dose range.

- Assessment of pharmacokinetic issues (ADME).
  The initials stand for **A**bsorption, **D**istribution, **M**etabolism, and **E**limination.

- Trials comprised of a small number of healthy subjects under the age of 50. Studies are usually of short duration.

Phase II
Phase II involves:

- Determination of drug efficacy within safe dose range.

- Trials comprised of a small number of subjects with the disease state or condition.

- Comparison of safety information with Phase I results.

Phase III
Phase III involves:

- Crucial juncture of drug development.

- Huge financial and strategic commitment by the company.

- Dramatic increase in the number of studies and subjects, potentially involving thousands of patients in multiple study sites in many countries.

- Determination if drug is as effective or more effective than other drugs on the market.

- Continuation of drug safety analysis and discovering any potential drug interactions.

- Longest and most expensive clinical trial process.

Phase IV

Phase IV involves:

- What occurs after drug is marketed.

- Possible requirements by a regulatory body for final approval of a drug.

- Cost versus benefit analysis against competitor products for insurance providers.

- Safety data.

Medical Writing and Consulting

Having the writing skills to produce specific, accurate, and complete medical literature is a qualification that is coveted by many institutions. Therefore, another possible PPE for pharmacy candidates is with a medical writing and/or consulting firm. These companies focus on contract work with larger companies in need of generating or publishing literature, such as study results, conference abstracts, and symposium booklets. This PPE's focus will be on writing, although you may also develop presentation slide sets, abstracts, and posters. Additionally, you will gain in-depth knowledge of clinical trial design, biostatistics, and database retrieval.

Notes

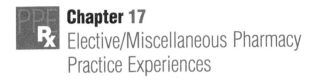

Chapter 17
Elective/Miscellaneous Pharmacy Practice Experiences

There are some PPE opportunities offered to pharmacy candidates that do not necessarily fall within any of the previously mentioned categories, but can be as challenging and rewarding as any of them.

PPE in Veterinary Medicine

During this PPE you will learn how drugs are used in veterinary practice, become acquainted with veterinary procedures, and gain an understanding of major differences between dosing across various species. It is important to note that many veterinary drug products have come about as a result of clinical trials investigating their use in humans. The preclinical stages of drug development always use multiple animal models to help determine basic characteristics of the medications, such as the ADME, mechanism of action, and toxicology (see Chapter 16). Therefore, by using animal models, you are not only studying a possible compound for human use, but for animal use as well.

PPEs with the U.S. Public Health Service

The U.S. Public Health Service Commissioned Corps (U.S. PHS) is comprised of more than 6,000 health care professionals dedicated to serving the nation and its health, disease prevention, and public health needs. Few may realize that the U.S. PHS is considered to be one of America's seven uniformed services. Furthermore, its highly skilled officers fill positions within the federal government as part of various agencies, departments, and divisions.

Officers of the U.S. PHS have a widely varied background in their roles, which include:

- Physicians

- Dentists

- Nurses

- Pharmacists

- Dietitians

- Engineers

- Environmental Health Officers

- Mental Health Workers

- Health Services Officers

- Scientists or Researchers

- Therapists

- Veterinarians

Where does a PHS officer actually practice pharmacy? As varied as the specialties, so too are the locations and agencies they may serve:

- Agency for Healthcare Research and Quality

- Agency for Toxic Substances and Disease Registry

- Centers for Disease Control and Prevention

- Food and Drug Administration

- Health Resources and Services Administration

- Centers for Medicare and Medicaid Services

- Indian Health Service

- National Institutes of Health

- Office of Public Health and Science

- Office of the Secretary, U.S. Department of Health and Human Services

- Substance Abuse and Mental Health Services Administration

- Office of the Assistant Secretary for Preparedness and Response

- Environmental Protection Agency

- Federal Bureau of Prisons

- National Oceanic and Atmospheric Administration

- National Park Service

- U.S. Department of Agriculture

- U.S. Department of Homeland Security

- Immigration and Customs Enforcement

- U.S. Coast Guard

- U.S. Marshals Service

This type of PPE, usually facilitated through the PHS Junior Commissioned Officer Student Training and Extern Program (JRCOSTEP), can be a very rigorous and demanding experience comprised of travel and difficult fluid situations. But it can also involve a tremendous amount of learning, teamwork, and camaraderie.

Notes

Appendices

The reference ranges given in these Appendices are general ones, commonly reported in medical literature and textbooks. During your PPEs, you should check with your supervisors at your particular site for the specific ranges used in patient and drug assessments. Different institutions may utilize different laboratory reference standards and practices.

Appendix A
Units of Measure and Conversions

Volume and Weight

Equivalents	Measures
1 g = 15.43 grains	1 fl oz = 30 mL
1 grain = 64.8 mg	1 cup (8 fl oz) = 240 mL
1 oz = 28.35 g	1 pint (16 fl oz) = 480 mL
1 lb = 453.6 g (0.4536 kg)	1 quart (32 fl oz) = 960 mL
1 kg = 2.2 lb	1 gallon (128 fl oz) = 3800 mL
1 fluid oz (fl oz) = 29.57 mL	1 teaspoon = 5 mL
1 pint (pt) = 473.2 mL	1 tablespoon = 15 mL
1 quart (qt) = 946.4 mL	1 oz = 30 g
	1 lb (16 oz) = 480 g
0.1 mg = 1/600 grain (gr)	15 grains = 1 g
0.12 mg = 1/500 gr	1 grain = 60 mg
0.15 mg = 1/400 gr	
0.2 mg = 1/300 gr	1 scruple = 20 grains (gr)
0.3 mg = 1/200 gr	60 grains = 1 dram
0.4 mg = 1/150 gr	8 drams = 1 ounce
0.5 mg = 1/120 gr	1 ounce = 480 grains
0.6 mg = 1/100 gr	16 ounces = 1 pound (lb)
0.8 mg = 1/80 gr	60 minims = 1 fluidram
1 mg = 1/65 gr	8 fluidrams = 1 fluid ounce
1 kg = 1000 g	
1 g = 1000 mg	
1 mg = 1000 μg	

Temperature
1°C = 1.8°F
1°F = 5/9°C
Fahrenheit to Centigrade or Celsius: (°F – 32) x 5/9 = °C
Centigrade or Celsius to Fahrenheit: (°C x 9/5) + 32 = °F

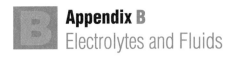

Appendix B
Electrolytes and Fluids

- Total body water (TBW) ~ 60% of body weight (kg) in males
  50% of body weight (kg) in females

- Ideal body weight (IBW)
  - Males = 50 kg + [2.3 kg x every inch of height >60 inches]
  - Females = 45.5 kg + [2.3 kg x every inch of height >60 inches]

- Body mass index (BMI) = kg / m^2

- Body surface area (BSA), m^2 = $\sqrt{\dfrac{\text{height(cm)} \times \text{weight(kg)}}{3600}}$

- Daily fluid requirements (maintenance, pediatrics)
  - 0-10 kg   100 mL/kg
  - 10-20 kg   additional 50 mL/kg
  - >20 kg   additional 20 mL/kg

Note: Use IBW in obese patients
Patients with fever: give an additional 10% for each 1° elevation

- Serum osmolality
  - mOsm/L = (2 x [Na^+]) + ([glucose in mg/dl] / 18) + (BUN / 2.8)

- Anion gap (AG) = Na^+ - (Cl^- + HCO_3^-)
  - Normal AG = 10-14 mEq/L

- Water Deficit = 0.6 x body weight (kg) x [1 – (140 / Na^+)]

- Free water deficit (FWD)
  - FWD = Normal TBW – Current TBW
    - Normal TBW (males) = lean body weight (kg) x 0.6 L/kg
    - Normal TBW (females) = lean body weight (kg) x 0.5 L/kg
    - Current TBW = normal TBW (140 / current [Na$^+$])

- Modification of Diet in Renal Disease (MDRD) = 186 x (SCr)$^{-1.154}$ x (Age)$^{-0.203}$ x (0.742 if female) x (1.210 if African-American)

- Estimated Creatinine Clearance = [Cl$_{cr}$(mL/min)]=
$$\frac{140 - \text{age}(y) \times \text{IBW (kg)}}{72 \times \text{Scr (mg/dL)}} \text{ x (0.85 if female)}$$

Composition of Intravenous Fluids Used for Volume Resuscitation

Fluids for intravenous replacement of extracellular volume or water deficit				
	[Na$^+$] (meq/L)	[Cl$^-$] (meq/L)	(mosm /L)	Other
0.9% NS	154	154	308	
5% D/0.9% NS	154	154	560	Glucose, 50 g/L
Lactated Ringers (LR)	130	109	273	K$^+$, Ca^{2+}, lactate[1]
5% D	0	0	252	Glucose, 50 g/L
0.45% NS	77	77	154	
5% D/0.45% NS	77	77	406	Glucose, 50 g/L

[1]K$^+$ 4 meq/L, Ca^{2+} 1.5 mEq/L, lactate 28 meq/L

Sodium Na$^+$ [135-145 mEq/L]
- Corrected Sodium = Na$^+_{measured}$ + [1.5 x (glucose – 150 divided by 100)]

Potassium K⁺ [3.5-5 mEq/L]

- Primarily an intracellular cation (only 2% is in serum)

- For each 1 mEq/L decrease in serum K^+, total body K^+ deficit is 150-200 mEq

- Hemolyzed blood samples can falsely elevate potassium levels

Potassium Deficit Treatment

	IV treatment for K⁺ deficit
RATE	Max rate = 10 mEq/h if not on cardiac monitor
	Max rate = 20 mEq/h if monitored
CONCENTRATION	Max for peripheral veins = 40 mEq/L
	Higher concentration (100 mEq/L) with central line

Calcium Ca²⁺ [8.5-10.5 mg/dl]

- Low albumin = low calcium level

- Corrected Serum Calcium for Albumin Level
  - [(Normal Alb – patient's Alb) x 0.8] + patient's measured total Ca^{2+}

Elemental Calcium Content

Calcium Salts		
Product	**Elemental Calcium Content**	**Route**
Ca-carbonate	20 mEq (400 mg)/g	PO
Ca-chloride	13.5 mEq (270 mg)/g	IV
Ca-gluconate	4.6 mEq (90 mg)/g	IV/PO
Ca-glubionate	3.2 mEq (64 mg)/g	PO

Magnesium Mg [1.5-2.0 mEq/L]
- 1 g Mg-sulfate = 8.1 mEq Mg

- IV Mg must be diluted and infused over several hours or IV push over several minutes

- IM is oftentimes painful

Phosphorus [3-4.5 mg/dl]
- Increased = renal insufficiency, laxative/enema abuse, tumor lysis syndrome, tissue necrosis, acidosis (respiratory, lactic), hypoparathyroidism

- Decreased = DKA, alcoholism, TPN, refeeding syndrome, burns, alkalosis (respiratory or metabolic), diarrhea, hyperparathyroidism

Chloride Cl [96-108 mEq/L]
- Cl Deficit = 0.4 x weight (kg) x (100 − measured Cl)

- Increased = dehydration, renal pathology, diabetes insipidus, head injury, respiratory alkalosis

- Decreased = GI losses, CHF, fluid overload, burns, excessive fluid loading

Bicarbonate HCO_3^- [22-28 mEq/L]
- HCO_3^- Deficit = (0.5 x kg) x (24 − HCO_3^- measured)

- Increased = compensatory respiratory acidosis, metabolic alkalosis

- Decreased = compensatory respiratory alkalosis, metabolic acidosis

Blood, Urea, Nitrogen BUN [6-20 mg/dl]

- End-product of protein-nitrogen metabolism

Serum Creatinine Scr [0.5-1.2 mg/dl]

- Increased = Acute and chronic renal failure, rhabdomyolysis

- Decreased = Decreased muscle mass (elderly)

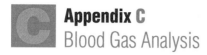

Appendix C
Blood Gas Analysis

Arterial Blood Gas (ABG) Analysis

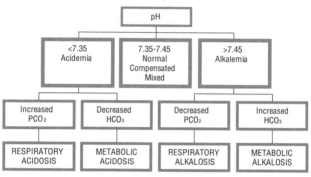

Metabolic Acidosis (normal AG)

HHARDUP = *underlying possible disorders*
- **H** Hypoaldosteronism
- **H** Hyperosmolar nonketotic coma
- **A** Acetazolamide
- **R** Renal Tubular Acidosis
- **D** Diarrhea
- **U** Ureterosigmoidostomy
- **P** Pancreatic Fistula

Metabolic Acidosis (elevated AG)

MUDPILES = *underlying possible disorders*
- **M** Methanol
- **U** Uremia
- **D** DKA
- **P** Poisons (paraldehyde, propylene glycol, phenformin)
- **I** Iron, INH (isoniazid)
- **L** Lactic Acidosis
- **E** Ethanol or ethylene glycol
- **S** Salicylates

Appendix D
Total Parenteral Nutrition

- If actual body weight (kg) > 120% IBW, use adjusted body weight (ABW)
  - ABW = [(Actual – IBW) x 0.2] + IBW

Caloric requirements	
Healthy individuals	Approx 25 kcal/kg/day
Malnourished or metabolically stressed	Approx 30 kcal/kg/day
Critically ill (i.e., ICU) or hypermetabolic	30-35 kcal/kg/day

Harris-Benedict Equation (estimating resting energy expenditure)	
Males	Kcal/d = 66 + [13.7 x wt(kg)] + [5 x ht(cm)] – (6.8 x age)
Females	Kcal/d = 665 + [9.6 x wt(kg)] + [1.8 x ht(cm)] – (4.7 x age)

Amino Acid (Protein) requirements	
Healthy individuals (maintenance)	0.8 g/kg/day
Moderate stress	1-1.5 g/kg/day
Hypermetabolic, severe stress	1.5-2 g/kg/day
Burns	2-2.5 g/kg/day
Renal failure	0.6-1 g/kg/day (no dialysis)
	1.2-2 g/kg/day (dialysis)
Hepatic failure	0.5-1.5 g/kg/day

Fluid requirements	
Adults – 30-35 mL/kg/day or daily fluid requirements calculation	
Children - daily fluid requirements calculation	

- 0-10 kg   100 mL/kg
- 10-20 kg   additional 50 mL/kg
- >20 kg   additional 20 mL/kg

Caloric conversions	
1 gram dextrose = 3.4 kcal	
1 gram amino acid (protein) = 4 kcal	
1 gram dietary fat = 9 kcal	
Intralipid (IV lipid emulsion; IVLE)	10% = 1.1 kcal/mL
	20% = 2 kcal/mL
	30% = 3 kcal/mL

Initiating electrolytes in TPN	
Na	1-3 mEq/kg/day
K	1-2 mEq/kg/day
PO_4	7-10 mMol/1000 kcal
Ca	0.1-0.3 mEq/kg/day (4.6 mEq is convenient)
Mg	0.3-0.45 mEq/kg/day (8.1 mEq is convenient)
Cl	1-3 mEq/kg/day
Acetate	0.5-3 mEq/kg/day

- Additional elements
  - Zinc 5 mg (wound healing)
  - Chromium 10 mcg
  - Copper 1 mcg
  - Selenium 80 mcg (wound healing)
  - MVI (multivitamin)

- Other drugs that may be added include heparin, insulin, H_2-blockers (famotidine)

  Note: In renal failure – do NOT give any K or PO_4

Example
60 kg male in moderate stress requiring TPN

1. 60 kg x 35 mL/kg/day = 2000 mL (2 L)

2. 60 kg x 30 kcal/kg/day = 1800 kcal

3. 60 kg x 1.2 g/kg/day amino acids (protein) = 72 g
   (protein x 4 kcal/g = 288 kcal)

4. 10% IVLE at 500 mL = 550 kcal
   (approximately 31% of total kcal)

5. 2000 mL – 500 mL = 1500 mL

6. 1800 kcal – 550 kcal IVLE = 1250 kcal

7. 1250 kcal – 288 kcal amino acids (protein) = 962 kcal
   (which is 283 g dextrose)

8. 283 g dextrose in 1500 mL = 19% Dextrose

9. 72 g amino acids (protein) in 1500 mL = 4.8%
   Amino Acids (Protein)

TPN order

19% Dextrose; 4.8% Amino Acids (Protein) running at 63
mL/h (1500 mL)

10% IVLE running at 21 mL/h (500 mL)

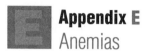

Appendix E
Anemias

Microcytic Anemia

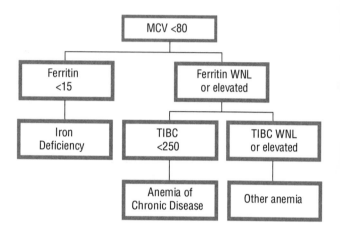

Normocytic Anemia

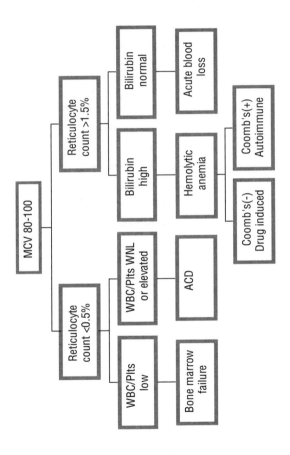

Macrocytic Anemia

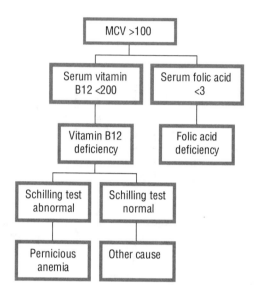

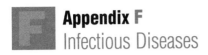

Appendix F
Infectious Diseases

Possible anatomic and physiologic correlations with a true infection:

1. Increased WBC (left shift; bands)

2. Hemodynamics
   a. Increased HR and cardiac output (CO)
   b. Decreased BP

3. Fever may be absent in overwhelming infections (sepsis)

4. Metabolic acidosis predominance

5. Hyperglycemia

6. Mental status changes

7. Respiratory distress

8. Coagulation disorders (i.e., increased PT, PTT)

Aerobic Gram Positive (Clusters)

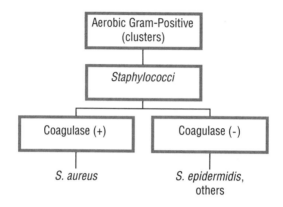

Aerobic Gram Positive (Chains)

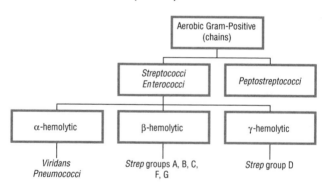

Aerobic Gram Negative (Rods)

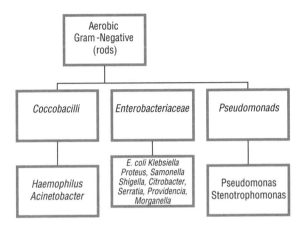

Anaerobes

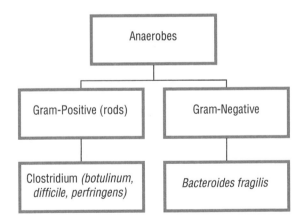

Appendix G
Therapeutic Range of Common Drug Level Assays

Drug	Therapeutic Range
Amantadine (trough)	300 ng/ml
Amikacin	
(trough)	1-8 mg/L
(peak)	20-30 mg/L
Amiodarone	0.5-2.5 mg/L
Amitriptyline	75-175 ng/ml
Amoxapine	200-500 ng/ml
Amrinone	1.5-4 mg/L
Bretylium	0.5-1.5 mg/L
Bupropion	25-100 ng/ml
Carbamazepine	4-12 mg/L
Chloramphenicol (peak)	10-20 mg/L
Chlorpromazine	50-300 ng/ml
Clomipramine	80-100 ng/ml
Cyclosporine	100-200 ng/ml (whole blood)
	50-300 ng/ml (plasma)
Digitoxin	9-25 mg/L
Digoxin	0.8-2 ng/ml
Disopyramide	2-8 mg/L
Doxepin	110-250 ng/ml
Flecainide (trough)	0.2-1 mg/L
Fluphenazine	0.13-2.8 ng/ml
Gentamicin	
(trough)	0.5-2 mg/L
(peak)	6-10 mg/L
Haloperidol	5-20 ng/ml
Hydralazine	100 ng/ml
Imipramine	50-200 ng/ml

continued on page 137

continued from page 136

Drug	Therapeutic Range
Kanamycin	
(trough)	5-10 mg/L
(peak)	20-25 mg/L
Lidocaine	1.5-6 mg/L
Lithium	0.6-1.2 mEq/L
Maprotiline	200-300 ng/ml
Mexiletine	0.5-2 mg/L
Netilmicin	
(trough)	0.5-2 mg/L
(peak)	6-10 mg/L
Nortriptyline	50-150 ng/ml
Perphenazine	0.8-2.4 ng/ml
Phenobarbital	10-40 mg/L
Phenytoin	10-20 mg/L
Primidone	4-12 mg/L
Procainamide	4-8 mg/L
Propranolol	50-200 ng/ml
Quinidine	2-6 mg/L
Streptomycin	
(trough)	<5 mg/L
(peak)	15-30 mg/L
Theophylline	10-20 mg/ml
Thiothixene	2-57 ng/ml
Tobramycin	
(trough)	0.5-2 mg/L
(peak)	5-10 mg/L
Tocainide	4-10 mg/L
Trazodone	800-1600 ng/ml
Valproic Acid	40-100 mg/L
Vancomycin	
(trough)	5-15 µg /mL
(peak)	20-40 µg /mL
Verapamil	50-400 µg /L

Index

B

C

S

T